Quick Look Nursing:
Pain Management

Second Edition

MARGARET SAUL LACCETTI, PHD, RN, AOCN, ACHPN
Boston College
Boston, Massachusetts

MARY K. KAZANOWSKI, PHD, APRN, BC, CHPN
Saint Anselm College
Manchester, New Hampshire

JONES AND BARTLETT PUBLISHERS
Sudbury, Massachusetts
BOSTON   TORONTO   LONDON   SINGAPORE

World Headquarters
Jones and Bartlett Publishers
40 Tall Pine Drive
Sudbury, MA 01776
978-443-5000
info@jbpub.com
www.jbpub.com

Jones and Bartlett Publishers Canada
6339 Ormindale Way
Mississauga, Ontario L5V 1J2
Canada

Jones and Bartlett Publishers International
Barb House, Barb Mews
London W6 7PA
United Kingdom

Jones and Bartlett's books and products are available through most bookstores and online booksellers. To contact Jones and Bartlett Publishers directly, call 800-832-0034, fax 978-443-8000, or visit our website, www.jbpub.com.

Substantial discounts on bulk quantities of Jones and Bartlett's publications are available to corporations, professional associations, and other qualified organizations. For details and specific discount information, contact the special sales department at Jones and Bartlett via the above contact information or send an email to specialsales@jbpub.com.

The authors, editor, and publisher have made every effort to provide accurate information. However, they are not responsible for errors, omissions, or for any outcomes related to the use of the contents of this book and take no responsibility for the use of the products and procedures described. Treatments and side effects described in this book may not be applicable to all people; likewise, some people may require a dose or experience a side effect that is not described herein. Drugs and medical devices are discussed that may have limited availability controlled by the Food and Drug Administration (FDA) for use only in a research study or clinical trial. Research, clinical practice, and government regulations often change the accepted standard in this field. When consideration is being given to use of any drug in the clinical setting, the health care provider or reader is responsible for determining FDA status of the drug, reading the package insert, and reviewing prescribing information for the most up-to-date recommendations on dose, precautions, and contraindications, and determining the appropriate usage for the product. This is especially important in the case of drugs that are new or seldom used.

Production Credits
Executive Editor: Kevin Sullivan
Acquisitions Editor: Emily Ekle
Acquisitions Editor: Amy Sibley
Editorial Assistant: Patricia Donnelly
Production Editor: Karen Ferreira
Associate Marketing Manager: Ilana Goddess
Cover Illustrator: Cara Judd
Cover Layout Artist: Tim Dziewit
Composition: Shawn Girsberger
Manufacturing and Inventory Control Supervisor: Amy Bacus
Printing and Binding: Malloy, Inc.
Cover Printing: Malloy, Inc.

Library of Congress Cataloging-in-Publication Data
Laccetti, Margaret Saul.
 Pain management / Margaret Saul Laccetti, Mary K. Kazanowski. — 2nd ed.
  p. ; cm. — (Quick look nursing)
 Rev. ed. of: Pain / Mary K. Kazanowski, Margaret Saul Laccetti. c2002.
 Includes bibliographical references and index.
 ISBN-13: 978-0-7637-4686-5
 1. Pain—Nursing. I. Kazanowski, Mary K. II. Kazanowski, Mary K. Pain. III. Title. IV. Series.
 [DNLM: 1. Pain—nursing. WY 160.5 L129p 2008]
 RT87.P35L33 2008
 616'.0472—dc22
                    2007038753

6048
Printed in the United States of America
12 11 10 09 08   10 9 8 7 6 5 4 3 2 1

Once again, this is dedicated to my men:
Tony, Andy, and Benjamin.
You are my life, my loves, and my reasons for being.

Margaret Saul Laccetti, PhD, RN, AOCN, ACHPN

I dedicate this book to all the patients and family caregivers
who have taught me so much about the experience of pain.

Mary Kazanowski, PhD, APRN, BC, CHPN

CONTENTS

ACKNOWLEDGMENTS

Thank you to all of the patients, families, students, and fellow healthcare professionals who continue to teach me how magical it is to be able to care for others.

Margaret Saul Laccetti PhD, RN, AOCN, ACHPN

I would like to acknowledge my colleagues in hospice who have taught me so much about the treatment of pain. I would also like to thank my husband, Glenn, for his support in this effort.

Mary Kazanowski, PhD, APRN, BC, CHPN

ABOUT THE AUTHORS

Margaret Saul Laccetti, PhD, RN, AOCN, ACHPN, is an assistant professor at Boston College. She is also an advanced practice nurse whose practice includes palliative care and caring for patients and families during cancer therapy.

Mary K. Kazanowski, PhD, APRN, BC, CHPN, is a professor in the Nursing Department at Saint Anselm College in Manchester, New Hampshire. She teaches medical–surgical nursing and community nursing. She is also a palliative care/hospice nurse at VNA Hospice of Manchester and Southern New Hampshire, and a Nurse Practitioner at the Wellstone House in Raymond, New Hampshire.

INTRODUCTION

Pain, defined as an unpleasant sensory or emotional experience arising from actual or potential tissue damage, is one of the most common reasons a patient interacts with a healthcare professional. It is experienced by individuals across the lifespan, and all along the trajectory of illness. Even otherwise healthy individuals may experience pain, as a warning system or protective mechanism. It is a subjective symptom; experienced by the patient, pain may occur with no visible objective signs or symptoms.

There are multiple and varied causes of pain. The experience can be related to trauma, stress, surgery, illness, hormonal changes, childbirth, inflammation, and ischemia. Manifestations of pain can be inconsistent, varying with the cause, site, and type of pain, as well as with patient-related variables. These variables can include physiologic, psychosocial, and cultural elements. Developmental or age-related physical changes, like myelination in infants or decreases in peripheral sensation in elder adults, may interfere with pain as a protective mechanism. Cognitive development, discussed later in this book, also affects the experience of pain. Cognitive impairment may reduce the patient's ability to express pain, resulting in undertreatment. Anxiety, fear, or identification of pain with serious illness may exacerbate a patient's pain experience. Family perceptions of pain or the meaning of the pain may also alter the experience or the patient's way of expressing or describing pain. Gender, ethnicity, socioeconomic status, access to heath care, and previous painful episodes all affect pain.

Frequently, severe pain that restricts activity or otherwise interferes with daily living is the precipitating factor for seeking out medical care. When daily living is not seriously affected, self-treatment for pain is a common choice. When self-care is not successful, medical care is an alternative.

Due to the complex nature of pain, providing relief is a challenging and multifaceted undertaking. Pain management is an ongoing process. It is frequently a negotiation between patient and healthcare provider. A comprehensive pain assessment is an essential step in designing interventions appropriate for each specific instance of pain. A plan of care must be constructed and implemented for each individual. Then, evaluation and modification of the plan will promote optimal pain management. In addition to considering patient-specific factors, a variety of management options should be considered and incorporated, including both pharmacologic and nonpharmocologic methods, as appropriate.

To be adequately prepared, healthcare professionals must pursue continued education regarding multiple methods of assessing and managing pain. In addition, personal biases, cultural elements, and financial considerations are important aspects included in plans for pain management.

The Joint Commission has identified pain as the fifth vital sign, an element necessary to assess in evaluating any patient's state of health. Historically, pain has been inappropriately managed or under-managed in the American healthcare system. A primary reason for this is fear of narcotic addiction. Through developing an understanding of the mechanics of the pain phenomenon, as well as of the pharmacology of medications, healthcare professionals will improve pain management. Incorporating nonpharmacological methods will add to the development of new and innovative strategies to relieve or prevent pain.

This text can be used to enhance the healthcare professional's ability to assess and manage pain competently. It will allow students and both new and experienced professionals to review the causes and physiology of pain, implications of developmental stages, age, and physical and psychosocial aspects of pain management. Both pharmacologic and non-pharmocologic methods of managing pain are presented and reviewed, in hopes that both will be of use in caring for the patients and families experiencing pain. Finally, selected pain experiences are used to illustrate assessment, management, and evaluation measures. It is the hope of both authors that this information will be useful in assessing, managing, and preventing pain as an integral part of health care.

References

Acute Pain Management Guideline Panel. (1992). *Acute pain management: Operative or medical procedures and trauma. AHCPR Pub No. 92-0032.* Rockville, MD: Agency for Health Care Policy and Research, Public Health Service, US Department of Health and Human Services.

Finely, G. A., McGrath, P., & Chambers, C.T. (2006). *Brining pain relief to children: Treatment approaches.* Totowa, NJ: Humana Press.

International Association for the Study of Pain. (2005). *Core curriculum for professional education in pain* (3rd ed.). Retrieved March 8, 2006, from http://www.iasp-pain.org/CoreCurriculumThirdEdition.htm

International Association for the Study of Pain. (2006). *Online curriculum on pain for nursing.* (2nd ed.). Retrieved March 8, 2006, from http://www.iasp-pain.org/NursingCurriculum2006.pdf

Joint Commission on the Accreditation of Health Care Organizations. *Pain standards.* Available at www.jcaho.org. Accessed 27 November 2007.

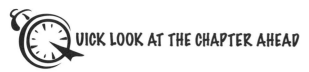

QUICK LOOK AT THE CHAPTER AHEAD

Pain is a subjective symptom experienced by individuals for a wide variety of reasons. Pain can be acute or chronic. Manifestations of pain can be inconsistent, varying with the cause, site and type of pain, as well as with patient-related variables.

Physiology of pain includes both the central nervous system (CNS) and the peripheral nervous system (PNS), mediated through a variety of chemical substances called neurotransmitters. Pain management includes methods addressing both the CNS and the PNS.

Different types of pain include superficial, visceral, somatic, neuropathic and pain resulting from metabolic need or metabolic excess.

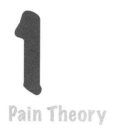

1

Pain Theory

TERMS
- [ ] acute pain
- [ ] central nervous system
- [ ] chronic pain
- [ ] depression
- [ ] intermittent claudication
- [ ] neuropathic pain
- [ ] neurotransmitters
- [ ] nociceptors
- [ ] objective
- [ ] pain
- [ ] peripheral arterial disease
- [ ] peripheral nervous system
- [ ] phantom pain
- [ ] prostaglandins
- [ ] referred pain
- [ ] subjective
- [ ] superficial pain
- [ ] visceral pain

CASE STUDY

Ms. P., a 27-year-old married woman, comes to the emergency department of a local community hospital complaining of severe pain in her back and right flank. She is pale and nauseated, and her skin is warm and dry. Skin turgor is poor. She appears dehydrated. On assessment, she localizes her pain in the right flank as well as in the central portion of her back. It is unrelieved by changing position. Prior to coming to the hospital, she attempted to relieve the back pain through use of a heating pad. This was not successful.

 ## PAIN: A SUBJECTIVE SYMPTOM

Pain is a universally experienced phenomenon. It is **subjective**, a perception of the individual. Pain has been described as being just what the individual experiencing it says it is. Being a subjective experience, severity, duration, and meaning are determined by the individual. Pain is characterized by some **objective** signs and symptoms; however, it cannot be assumed that all people will exhibit these objective signs as a part of the pain experience. Clients describe the experience as acute or chronic discomfort. In descriptive assessment, the type and severity of the pain are often characterized as agony, pulling, pressure, burning, stinging, searing, stabbing, dull, aching, and so on. More than one type, sensation, or source of pain may coexist for one client at one time. It is a phenomenon that *must* be carefully assessed to plan interventions.

There are multiple and varied causes of pain. The experience can be related to trauma (major or minor), stress, surgery, illness, hormonal changes, childbirth, inflammation, and ischemia. Episodes of pain occur in the client in clinical as well as nonclini-

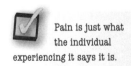
Pain is just what the individual experiencing it says it is.

cal situations. Frequently, severe pain that restricts activity or otherwise interferes with daily living is the precipitating factor for seeking medical care. When daily living is not seriously affected, self-treatment for pain is a common choice. When self-care is not successful, medical care may become an alternative choice.

Acute Pain or Chronic Pain?

Acute pain usually occurs with an identifiable precipitating factor. It varies in type and severity, and it may be constant or intermittent. Description of pain as *acute* does not refer to severity; rather, it describes the time period in which the particular pain is experienced. Episodes of pain that are resolved in less than 6 months are considered to be acute. **Chronic pain** refers to episodes that take more than 6 months to resolve. This does not presume that relief for acute or chronic pain cannot be successfully initiated within that time frame. Rather, it indicates that the cause or precipitating factor is identified and successfully eliminated or controlled before or after a 6-month time span.

Symptoms of acute and chronic pain frequently differ on objective assessment (**Figure 1-1**). The client in acute pain more closely fits the stereotypical or traditional picture of pain. Activities such as grimacing, splinting, guarding, moaning, or crying are often observed, although they may not directly correlate with severity. The client with acute pain usually exhibits a change in routine level of activity, with progressively severe pain preventing successful completion of activities of daily living (ADLs). The client may become anxious or agitated with acute pain. This type of

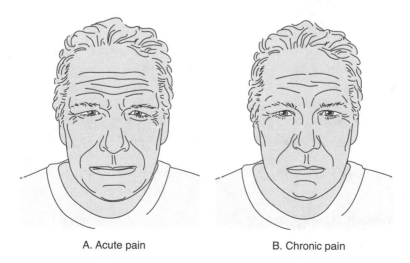

A. Acute pain   B. Chronic pain

Figure 1-1 A. Acute pain denoted by obvious distress, autonomic symptoms, grimacing, and crying. B. Chronic pain denoted by not-so-obvious distress and flattened affect.

pain is seen as predictable. It can usually be controlled or eliminated; it is expected and self-limiting with the cause or precipitating factor. Physical assessment of the client in acute pain usually reveals an increase in vital signs, specifically pulse and respirations (hyperactivity of the autonomic nervous system). Blood pressure may be seen to either increase or decrease, with a decrease indicating potential for shock. The client in acute pain is frequently pale and diaphoretic.

 Symptoms of acute and chronic pain frequently differ on objective assessment.

Chronic pain manifests quite differently. The client does not look like someone in pain by traditional standards. The chronicity of the painful experience has caused the expression of pain to differ, especially in relation to restrictions with ADLs. Chronic pain is not predictable and has no anticipated end point. It is frequently undertreated because

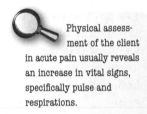

Physical assessment of the client in acute pain usually reveals an increase in vital signs, specifically pulse and respirations.

the healthcare provider does not assess the client as being in significant pain. There is commonly no remarkable deviation in vital signs or other observable physiological parameters upon assessment. Fatigue and social isolation are common sequelae of chronic pain. Rather than grimacing or agitation, the client in pain may exhibit slack facial features, reduced activity levels, and a flattened affect. **Depression** may accompany chronic pain. It is essential for the healthcare provider to recognize, acknowledge, and treat chronic pain as the client describes it. Treatment of chronic pain includes long-term use of prescribed interventions. With this in mind, interventions should be cost effective or affordable, easy to understand and practice, readily available, and believable. By considering these factors for each individual client, compliance with treatment will be more commonly assured. It is also important to frequently reassess the chronic pain client.

 # PHYSIOLOGY OF PAIN

The sensation of pain involves both the **peripheral** and **central nervous systems**. It is primarily a warning signal to avoid injury. Response to pain is often reflexive. The central nervous system mediates other responses.

Specialized nerve cells, called *nociceptors*, are sensory receptors found in skin, muscle, viscera, and connective tissue. These nerve cells respond to stimulation caused by thermal, mechanical, or chemical injury. The response is release of chemical mediators including **prostaglandins**. The chemical mediators cause the nociceptor to "fire," carrying the pain impulse to the spinal cord. These impulses travel along afferent nerve fibers, either myelinated A-delta fibers or unmyelinated C fibers.

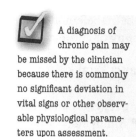

A diagnosis of chronic pain may be missed by the clinician because there is commonly no significant deviation in vital signs or other observable physiological parameters upon assessment.

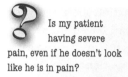

Is my patient having severe pain, even if he doesn't look like he is in pain?

Gate Control Theory

The gate control theory, first proposed by scientists in 1965, argues that pain is not transmitted directly from the spinal cord to the central nervous system. Rather, a complex nerve structure in the dorsal horns of the spinal cord can inhibit transmission of the pain message to the brain. These gates operate by means of various **neurotransmitters** including substance P and somatostatin. Prevention of transmission to the brain also prevents the recognized sensation of pain. The response to the injury is reflexive, and the source of the unpleasant stimulus is eliminated. The stimulus only becomes pain as it is sensed consciously.

Sensory information from various areas within the body may converge at spinal neurons. This convergence is responsible for the sensation of referred pain, the pain that is perceived in a part of the body other than where the injury or stimulus has originated. By utilizing the gates in the spinal dorsal horns, a variety of methods to 'close the gate' to painful stimuli are utilized to relieve or prevent pain.

TYPES OF PAIN

There is a wide variety of pain and pain sensations. The variety is a product of the multiple causes of pain as well as the unique responses to painful stimuli, especially the components of higher central nervous system responses. Pain, as discussed earlier, can be acute or chronic. Symptoms of these types differ, as do the potential interventions for control and relief. The emotional reaction of the client also changes in response to acuity or chronicity.

Superficial Pain

Superficial pain is extremely common across the lifespan. It is the result of stimulation of the most superficial nociceptors in cutaneous tissue, such as skin or mucous membranes. These areas are rich in afferent fibers, since one of their functions is to gather information about the world outside of the organism. Given the wealth of receptive nervous tissue in these areas, superficial pain can be experienced by the individual as quite severe or intense. Superficial or cutaneous pain may result from mechanical injury, such as scraping, abrasion, or compression (pinching the tissue). Thermal injury, including both heat and cold, is another cause of superficial pain. Finally, chemical injury causes this type of pain. It is frequently described in two distinct patterns: the first, with rapid, acute onset at the time of injury, is frequently a sharp piercing or stinging sensation; the second is cutaneous pain that arises well after the painful event and may be a deeper burning sensation that is longer-lasting and more difficult to relieve. It is easily localized by the client, who can usually identify the exact location as well as the precipitating event. Potential interventions may be local—such as the application of cold, heat, or pressure—or systemic. Superficial pain is not always accompanied by obvious signs of injury. When there is obvious injury, fear, anxiety, or other intense emotions may complicate the pain and the efforts to offer relief.

 Superficial pain is characterized in two distinct patterns: rapid, acute onset at the time of injury, consisting of a sharp piercing or stinging sensation, or cutaneous pain, occurring well after the painful event, consisting of a deep burning sensation that is longer-lasting and more difficult to relieve.

 Fear, anxiety, or other intense emotions may complicate pain management.

Visceral Pain

Pain that arises from stimulation of deeper nociceptors may be visceral (sometimes called organ pain) or somatic (structural pain). **Visceral pain** can arise in the thoracic, abdominal, pelvic, or cranial cavities. It is diffuse, poorly localized, and frequently difficult to identify with diagnosis.

Symptoms commonly associated with visceral pain are indicative of autonomic nervous system activity. They include pallor, diaphoresis, abdominal cramping, and diarrhea. There is often a significant increase in the client's blood pressure. Visceral pain may not come from the specific organ system where damage has occurred but may be caused by pressure or inflammation in surrounding tissues. One excellent example is abdominal pain accompanying intestinal disorders such as diverticulitis or colon cancer. The inside of the large intestine is poorly innervated with afferent fibers. As a matter of fact, patients with ostomies may have no sensation at the mucous membrane portion of the stoma, which is constructed from the interior of the large intestine. Rather, abdominal pain accompanying these illnesses may arise from stimulation of afferent fibers in the omentum or abdominal wall. Another source of painful stimuli is strong muscular contractions of hollow organs such as the stomach or bladder, resulting in visceral pain.

Visceral pain is described as deep, aching, cramping, or intense pressure. It is this type of pain that is frequently "referred" to other areas of the body. **Referred pain** is a sensation that actually arises in one organ system or area of the body but is perceived by the client to be occurring in another area (**Figure 1-2**).

One example of referred pain is back pain as part of the symptom set of cholecystitis. Sensation of pain at an area other than its source may complicate timely diagnosis or delay the client's attempts to access medical care. The client experiencing back pain associated with cholecystitis may first use self-care methods such as heat, massage, and over-the-counter nonsteroidal anti-inflammatory drugs (NSAIDs) to manage the pain.

Referred pain arises in one organ system or area of the body but is perceived to be occurring in another area.

Somatic Pain

Somatic or structural pain is more easily localized by the client and is frequently associated with trauma or activity. It may arise in muscles, joints, bones ligaments, tendons, or fascia. The client's description of the pain may vary from sharp and severe to dull and achy. Somatic pain may be constant or intermittent, and the client often relates it to activity or positioning. Structural tissues may stimulate afferent nerve fibers because of traumatic injury such as tearing or crushing. Afferent fibers may also be stimulated by pressure, such as the result of tumor invasion,

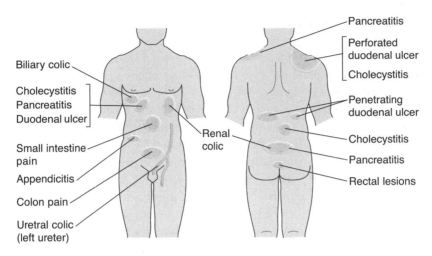

Figure 1-2 Common pathways of referred pain as they relate to an underlying abnormality.

swelling, venous congestion, or chemical irritation, as in rheumatoid arthritis. Deeper somatic pain is often more poorly localized and may be experienced and reported by the client as referred pain. Clients will frequently attempt self-care measures to relieve somatic pain. This type of pain may indicate conditions that are progressive. Early intervention in these cases can prevent further injury or complications.

Pain as the Result of Metabolic Need or Metabolic Excess

Pain is often the result of metabolic need or metabolic excess in clients with vascular disease or vascular compromise. Atherosclerosis is the most common form of vascular disease. Risk factors for atherosclerosis include hypertension, hyperlipidemia, obesity, inactivity, smoking, and heredity. Clearly, many of these risk factors can be positively managed through selected nursing interventions. Atherosclerosis may affect arterial or venous structures. Symptoms and treatment modalities of arterial or venous vascular disease differ greatly. Arterial vascular disease causes pain as the result of insufficient oxygen and nutrients in muscle or organ systems. Such pain is called *ischemic* pain. Ischemic pain is an excellent early warning system, since it is experienced even when no overt damage occurs. Arterial vascular disease occurs in central, coronary, or peripheral circulation. Central circulation, including large vessels such as the abdominal or thoracic portions of the aorta or the carotid arteries, may be the source of pain resulting from insufficient blood flow to organs or organ systems such as the kidneys or brain. Pain may also be the result of aneurysm formation in these vessels, compromising blood flow beyond the aneurysm. Pain also occurs as the result of direct pressure on surrounding tissues and organs when the aneurysm is quite large. Severe pain is a clinical indicator of dissection, or rupture of an aneurysm, which is a potentially life-threatening event.

 Ischemic pain is a hallmark of impending damage.

Coronary artery disease accounts for a very large portion of chest pain reported to healthcare providers. Narrowing of the coronary arteries by atherosclerotic plaque formation, embolism, or vasoconstriction 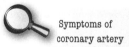 **What are the client's risk factors for vascular disease?** interrupts blood flow to the coronary muscle, often resulting in characteristic chest pain symptoms. These include a sense of crushing pressure, severe pain radiating to the left arm or jaw accompanied by diaphoresis, nausea, shortness of breath, and weakness. Less common symptoms may include radiating pain to the right arm, abdominal pain, or aching sensations in the left jaw, neck, and/or arm. This pain is called *angina*. It indicates a need for oxygen to the coronary muscle but does not necessarily indicate a destructive process. When overt damage occurs to the coronary muscle, this is called a *myocardial infarction* (MI). Anginal pain may be relieved with rest, which decreases the oxygen deficit. It may also respond to administration of oxygen or the use of vasodilators or medications such as nitroglycerin. Opioids are not used to relieve pain during an attack of angina but may be administered to the client who has experienced an MI for management of pain as well as to reduce anxiety.

Symptoms of coronary artery disease include a sense of crushing pressure, severe pain radiating to the left arm or jaw accompanied by diaphoresis, nausea, shortness of breath, and weakness. Less common symptoms may include radiating pain to the right arm, abdominal pain, or aching sensations in the left jaw, neck, and/or arm.

Peripheral arterial disease may be chronic or acute. The acute form occurs as the result of diminished peripheral circulation as the result of trauma, hypovolemia, or emboli. Pain is usually well localized and severe, with location depending on which arteries are blocked. Treatment includes treating the cause of the blockage, increasing oxygen transport to the area, and preventing damage below the blockage. Opioids may be used in conjunction with other treatment modalities to relieve the pain. *Heat should never be used to promote comfort when arterial compromise is suspected.* The application of superficial heat to the area results in increased metabolism. This increases the need for oxygen, exacerbates the oxygen deficit, and can result in organ or tissue damage.

 Heat should never be used to promote comfort when arterial compromise is suspected.

Chronic peripheral arterial disease occurs as the result of progressive narrowing of the peripheral arteries and arterioles. Onset is usually subtle and insidious. The hallmark symptom is called **intermittent claudication**, a pain that occurs with exercise and is relieved with rest. It is related to the muscle's oxygen deficit with exercise. This pain is usually reported by the client as severe, occurring in the calf. It may radiate to the thigh and buttocks. When the activity is stopped, the pain slowly recedes. Elevation of the legs does not reduce the pain; rather, keeping the legs dependent uses gravity to promote arterial blood flow. Clients with severe peripheral arterial disease report night pain, particularly a severe pain in the calf, which that may radiate to the thigh and buttocks, that wakes them from sleep. This pain is the result of oxygen deficit related to the reduced cardiac output during sleep and to the position of the client's legs (usually elevated in the bed). The client will report that the pain is usually resolved by dangling the legs over the side of the bed or sitting with both feet on the floor. Some clients report that this pain is so severe and frequent that they are forced to sleep in a chair, with their legs dependent. Several interventions are appropriate to promote pain relief. Clients may self-medicate with aspirin or NSAIDs. Vasodilators sometimes help. Maintaining the legs in a dependent position may prevent or relieve the pain. A supervised program of progressive exercise to the point of pain may promote formation of collateral

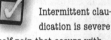 Intermittent claudication is severe calf pain that occurs with exercise and is relieved with rest as a result of the muscle's oxygen deficit with exercise.

 Severe peripheral arterial disease can lead to a severe nighttime pain in the calf that may radiate to the thigh and buttocks, the result of oxygen deficit related to the reduced cardiac output during sleep and to the position of the client's legs (usually elevated in the bed).

circulation. The goals of these interventions are to promote relief and prevent tissue damage. Remember to teach clients never to use superficial heat in an attempt to relieve this pain. Many clients with severe disease elect to have surgical revascularization procedures such as arterial bypass.

 Treating pain of peripheral arterial disease may include a supervised program of progressive exercise to the point of pain to promote formation of collateral circulation.

Clients with peripheral narrowing of the veins from disease, compression, thrombosis, or embolization also report pain. This pain may be deep, burning, or aching, can be constant or intermittent, and is commonly well localized. The pain may be the result of a build-up of toxins in the surrounding tissues that are not adequately removed through venous circulation. It may result from inflammation or may occur because of edematous pressure on surrounding tissues. Edema occurs when valves in the peripheral veins become incompetent, allowing the column of blood to fall back with gravity, distending the veins. Valves are frequently destroyed by deposits of atherosclerotic plaque or the formation of thromboses. Changes in pressure gradients promote the flow of fluid into the extravascular spaces. Clients with pain as the result of peripheral venous disease do not relate it to activity. Relief may be promoted through elevation or movement. Inflammatory processes that accompany thrombosis may be relieved through the use of anti-inflammatory drugs such as NSAIDs, application of superficial heat, and elevation.

 Pain from peripheral venous disease is not related to activity, and is the result of a build-up of toxins in the surrounding tissues, inflammation, or edematous pressure on surrounding tissues.

Pain from peripheral *arterial* disease occurs with activity and is relieved by rest; pain from peripheral *venous* disease is not related to activity and is relieved with elevation or movement.

Neuropathic Pain

Neuropathic pain, also called neuroleptic pain, differs from the types of pain previously discussed. Rather than pain that occurs as the result of information transmitted from tissue or organs via nociceptors, neuropathic pain results from damage to the peripheral or central nervous system. Stimulation of the nerves is not necessary for the client to report experiencing pain. Methods of stimulation that were not painful prior to the nerve damage may now be reported to be exquisitely painful. The reported sensations and methods for relief are very different from nociceptor pain. The pain can be mild to very severe and is frequently described as a burning, searing sensation. It is poorly localized and does not respond to conventional interventions. Neuropathic pain is commonly continuous rather than intermittent. It may be accompanied by paresthesias, sensations of heat or cold, tingling, numbness, or paralysis. As a result of the damage to the nerves, neuropathic pain often becomes a chronic symptom that can be seriously debilitating. Because the damage may not be visible and conventional relief methods are often useless, clients with this type of pain are sometimes considered malingerers, complainers, or noncompliant. Finding relief for these clients is a challenge to healthcare professionals. Positional changes or cutaneous or transcutaneous stimulation may offer some relief. Use of opioids almost always fails to help. Antiseizure medications such as phenytoin (Dilantin) have been used with good effect.

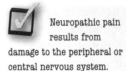 Neuropathic pain results from damage to the peripheral or central nervous system.

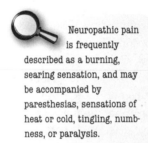 Neuropathic pain is frequently described as a burning, searing sensation, and may be accompanied by paresthesias, sensations of heat or cold, tingling, numbness, or paralysis.

Nursing interventions for management of chronic pain, including relaxation, visualization, distraction, prioritizing, and pacing activities, are valuable to the client with neuropathic pain. Medical interventions may include nerve blocks and surgery.

 Neuropathic pain is not relieved with conventional methods, such as opioids.

Phantom Pain

One specific form of neuropathic pain occurs after an amputation. This is called **phantom pain**. It is pain experienced by the client in the portion of the body that has been amputated, but it is not a function of the client's imagination. Phantom pain arises from damage to nerve fibers at the stump. The type of pain varies widely but is often accompanied by sensations similar to other types of neuropathic pain, including burning sensations and paresthesias. The client may also report sensations that feel as though the missing limb is in an uncomfortable or cramped position. Nursing interventions for phantom pain include teaching about this very real phenomenon. Fear, anxiety, misunderstanding, and denial of or reluctance to report the pain inhibit attempts at providing relief. Relaxation, visualization, and having the client imagine moving the missing area into a more comfortable position are sometimes helpful. Stimulation at the stump may also relieve some of the phantom sensation. Another alternative to promote relief includes having the client move or massage the opposite body part (the right foot if the left foot is missing). Anti-inflammatory medications are sometimes helpful in the acute stages following the amputation. Opioids are limited in their effect. Other interventions for neuropathic pain are helpful in relieving phantom pain.

 Phantom pain arises from damage to nerve fibers at the area of amputation. Although frequently associated with limb amputations, it is frequently experienced by women after mastectomy.

CASE STUDY REVISITED

After a variety of diagnostic tests, it is determined that the source of Mrs. P.'s pain is a kidney stone. She is admitted to the hospital in preparation for hydration and pain management. Before she is transported to the surgical inpatient unit, an intravenous (IV) line is placed for hydration. The nurse who is to start the IV first uses a topical anesthetic on the area to reduce the superficial pain of inserting the needle.

VARIABLES AFFECTING PAIN

A multitude of variables may affect the pain experienced by the client. They can include mood, anxiety, fear, stress, powerlessness, anger, reluctance to discuss pain, shame, sleeplessness, fatigue, and culture. These variables affect the expression of pain, as well as its severity and meaning in the client's life. For many of these variables, a circuitous pattern may be established, with pain enhancing the variable while the variable exacerbates the pain.

 Depression, mood, anxiety, fear, stress, powerlessness, anger, reluctance to discuss pain, shame, sleeplessness, fatigue, and culture affect the expression of pain, as well as its severity and meaning in the client's life.

Clients in pain frequently suffer from depression, which may range from a simple case of the blues to a long-term clinical depression warranting medical intervention. The depression may be related to the experience of pain itself or may revolve around issues such as diagnosis, immobility, change in role, or body image changes. Depression may also be a variable that exists independent of the pain experience, yet is an exacerbating factor. The client who is depressed may have increased experience of pain. This client may have difficulty in reporting pain, seeking relief, or compliance with a pain relief regimen. Although depression is often associated with chronic pain, it may be a factor for the client in acute pain as well. Symptoms of depression include flattened affect, reported feelings of sadness, decreased pleasure or interest, changes in appetite and sex drive, and sleep disturbances. Assessing for and offering interventions for depression will result in a greater potential for optimal pain relief.

Fear, anxiety, and increased stress may exacerbate pain as well as introduce barriers to pain relief. *Fear* is a sense of discomfort with a defined or specific stressor. It may be fear of tests, treatments or procedures, a diagnosis, or an outcome. Clients fear death, pain, and situations that are potentially painful. Many other specific items or ideas may be feared.

> Is the client in pain also suffering from depression? Is the depression being appropriately treated?

Fear can impede the client's ability or willingness to seek out diagnosis or treatment for pain. The client who fears needles will certainly be reluctant to use a pain relief option that involves intramuscular or subcutaneous injections. Not all fears are rational, obvious, or easily understood by the healthcare provider. Through careful and sensitive assessment, stressors that are feared may be identified. Once identified, they can be addressed and managed to enhance client comfort.

Anxiety is a sense of uneasiness or discomfort with no concrete causative factor or specific stressor. Given the more vague, global nature of anxiety, it is sometimes more difficult to manage. Anxiety, like fear, may present significant barriers to diagnosis and treatment. In addition, physiological changes may accompany anxiety, which cause or exacerbate pain. Increased muscular tension and metabolism are common symptoms of anxiety that can cause pain, such as the all-too-common tension-related headache. Muscular tension can also exacerbate existing pain syndromes. It can cause diagnostic or treatment-related procedures to be much more difficult and painful. A calm, professional attitude on the part of the caregiver is essential in helping the client to deal with anxiety. Privacy, a comfortable environment, minimal waiting time, and reduced cues to anxiety will also help. Relaxation techniques, guided imagery, music therapy, breathing exercises, and distraction are several other strategies for helping the client to reduce anxiety. Finally, adequate, clear information and direct instruction are useful in offering the anxious client intervention for pain. When someone is fearful or anxious, it is often difficult for him or her to listen, attend to a situation, and retain information. Concentration is a major effort for the client. Speak slowly, clearly, and repeat important information or instructions. Written, audiotaped, or videotaped information may be other methods of sharing information. Stress that is unrelated to the client's pain or medical condition can frequently lead to other anxieties or fears. Pain does not occur independently of the rest of the client's life. It is important to attempt to assess for other stressors to prevent their interference with pain management.

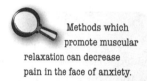

Methods which promote muscular relaxation can decrease pain in the face of anxiety.

Powerlessness is a sense that no action taken on the part of the individual will result in change. Powerlessness may be related to disease, diagnosis, or prognosis. A change in roles may force the client to relinquish decision-making, enhancing a sense of powerlessness. Situational powerlessness may occur in interactions between the client and healthcare providers when information is withheld or control is usurped by the healthcare team. It can also be related to lack of knowledge, physical disabilities, isolation, and chronicity of pain. The client who perceives himself to be powerless in pain relief presents a challenge similar to the client suffering from depression.

Anger is a powerful destructive force, using large amounts of energy to sustain. It is exhausting, and it presents a barrier to communication and pain relief. The client may be angry at something that is related to his or her illness or pain; however, the anger may be completely unrelated. Assisting the client to resolve anger will help to reduce barriers to pain relief.

Sleep disturbances and fatigue are often associated with pain. *Fatigue* is feeling tired unrelated to sleep or energy expended. It is not relieved by rest and can be severely debilitating. It is associated with multiple disease states including anemia, cancer, and depression. Fatigue is frequently related to chronic pain. It can be implicated in reducing the client's tolerance for pain as well as a barrier to seeking out intervention or being proactive in pain management. Pain is one primary reason for sleep disturbances. Certain pain medications, including opioids, may interfere with REM (rapid eye movement) stage sleep, reducing the benefits of the time spent sleeping. Sleep deprivation can affect the client's ability to deal with pain in similar ways to fatigue. It can also make it difficult for the client to concentrate and communicate effectively. Sleep deprivation can be resolved by identifying and correcting the causes.

 Fatigue can be related to either acute or chronic pain.

 Pain disrupts sleep; sleep deprivation exacerbates pain!

The client's cultural background may affect the way pain is experienced, manifested, reported, or described. It may determine the meaning of the pain in the client's life. Culture also determines the appropriateness of certain interventions. Finally, the culture of the client or caregiver can introduce certain biases into the pain intervention process. Culture may dictate how a client manifests his or her pain. It may also result in differences in manifestation between men and women. In some cultures, stoicism in the face of pain is required, inhibiting assessment and preventing intervention. In other cultures, especially in certain situations, pain is openly and verbally expressed. At times, these expressions may appear to the healthcare provider to be out of proportion with the perceived severity of the pain. It is important for the nurse not to allow biases or cultural differences to interfere with assessment or intervention.

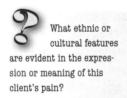 What ethnic or cultural features are evident in the expression or meaning of this client's pain?

CASE STUDY RESOLVED

Mrs. P.'s pain is well managed through use of a PCA (patient-controlled analgesia) pump. The PCA pump is discontinued 24 hours after admission, and her pain is then managed with an oral opioid and NSAID combination. With increased hydration, she passes the stone without any other intervention. She is discharged home after education on prevention of renal calculi is provided.

CHAPTER 1 · REVIEW QUESTIONS

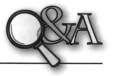

1. Pain can be best described as:
    A. An objective phenomenon, primarily characterized by observable signs and symptoms
    B. A symptom consistently seen with trauma or disease
    C. A subjective phenomenon, perceived by the individual and characterized by what the individual says it is
    D. A symptom that has no particular relation to the illness or trauma

2. When pain is severe and restricts or limits activities of daily living, the client will commonly:
    A. Self-medicate
    B. Seek out medical intervention
    C. Limit all social interactions
    D. Identify the precipitating factors before seeking relief

3. The client experiencing chronic pain:
    A. Exhibits crying, grimacing, and other classic symptoms
    B. Severely limits activities
    C. Is pale and diaphoretic
    D. May appear to have no observable symptoms

4. Common signs and symptoms associated with acute pain include:
    A. Increase in pulse and respiration, pallor, and either increase or decrease in blood pressure
    B. Ruddy complexion, bradycardia, and shortness of breath
    C. Decrease in pulse, respirations, and blood pressure
    D. Syncope and diaphoresis

5. The sensation of pain involves:
    A. The peripheral nervous system
    B. Both the peripheral and central nervous systems
    C. The autonomic nervous system
    D. The central nervous system

6. The gate control theory argues that:
   A. All pain sensations must be passed through a series of gates to be perceived and acted upon
   B. Gates that are active in transmitting messages of pain operate through the use of prostaglandins
   C. A complex structure in the dorsal horns of the spinal cord can inhibit the transmission of pain; the gate is then closed
   D. Only reflexive reactions occur in response to pain

7. One common example of pain that occurs as the result of metabolic need or excess is:
   A. Pain as the result of myocardial infarction
   B. Migraine headache
   C. Trauma-induced pain
   D. Labor

8. Intermittent claudication, the hallmark symptom of chronic peripheral arterial disease, is characterized by:
   A. Severe, unrelenting chest pain at night
   B. Pain in the legs that occurs with exercise and is relieved by rest
   C. Pain in the calf that occurs when legs are raised and is relieved by moving to a leg-dependent position
   D. Numbness, pain, and blanching of the fingers and toes

9. All of the following are characteristics of neuropathic pain except:
   A. Neuropathic pain is successfully relieved through the use of morphine
   B. Neuroleptic medications may be used in the treatment of neuropathic pain
   C. Neuropathic pain is more commonly persistent, rather than intermittent
   D. A particular type of neuropathic pain is phantom pain

10. A client's cultural background:
    A. Never affects the way pain is perceived or expressed
    B. Always presents a significant barrier to pain management
    C. May determine the appropriateness or acceptability of an intervention
    D. Is not useful in determining a plan of care for the client in pain

ANSWERS AND RATIONALES

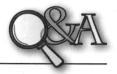

1. **C.** Pain is subjective, may have no observable manifestations, and should be recognized as being whatever the individual experiencing it says it is.

2. **B.** When pain limits normal activities, the client will seek medical intervention. If pain does not restrict activities or daily living, self-medication is usually attempted.

3. **D.** The client in chronic pain may have no observable traditional signs and symptoms of pain, yet may still be experiencing severe pain that needs intervention. It is more difficult for the nurse to assess.

4. **A.** Increase in pulse and respiration, pallor, and either increase or decrease in blood pressure are indicative of hyperactivity of the autonomic nervous system associated with acute pain.

5. **B.** Both the peripheral and central nervous systems are used in sensing pain.

6. **C.** Pain is not transmitted directly from the peripheral to the central nervous system, but through a gate or complex nervous structure in the dorsal horn of the spinal cord through various neurotransmitters including substance P and somatostatin.

7. **A.** The pain resulting from myocardial infarction is the product of oxygen deficit.

8. **B.** Pain that occurs with exercise and is relieved by rest is caused by oxygen deficit and lactic acid build-up in the calf muscles, relieved by rest and dangling the legs.

9. **A.** Opioids are rarely useful in the treatment of neuropathic pain.

10. **C.** A client's cultural background may determine if an intervention or the healthcare professional who offers the intervention is appropriate, acceptable, or useful for that particular client.

REFERENCES

Acute Pain Management Guideline Panel. (1992). *Acute pain management: operative or medical procedures and trauma. AHCPR Pub No. 92-0032.* Rockville, MD: Agency for Health Care Policy and Research, Public Health Service, U.S. Department of Health and Human Services.

Braun, C. A., & Anderson, C. M. (2007). *Pathophysiology: functional alterations in human health.* Philadelphia: Lippincott Williams & Wilkins.

International Association for the Study of Pain. (2005). *Core curriculum for professional education in pain* (3rd ed.). http/www.iasp-pain.org/CoreCurriculumThirdEdition.htm (accessed on 8 March 2006).

International Association for the Study of Pain. (2006). *Online curriculum on pain for nursing* (2nd ed.). http/www.iasp-pain.org/NursingCurriculum2006.pdf (accessed on 8 March 2006).

Karch, A. M. (2005). *2006 Lippincott's nursing drug guide.* Philadelphia: Lippincott Williams & Wilkins.

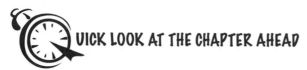

Using the nursing process, the nurse must be able to assess the client in order to identify pain as a problem. A comprehensive pain assessment is an essential step in designing interventions appropriate for each specific instance of pain. Streamlining the assessment process requires structure as well as innovation, especially in an attempt to reduce barriers to the assessment process. Pain is a primary barrier in the assessment process.

Developing a comprehensive pain history includes interviewing the client for a subjective history of pain, using a pain scale to rate intensity or severity. Investigating symptoms that accompany the pain and comorbidities that impact mood, habits, and ability to participate in activities of daily living is also essential. Physical assessment for pain involves identification of objective signs of pain. It is not the goal of the pain assessment to diagnose the cause of pain. A rapid head-to-toe assessment can identify contributing factors as well as barriers to assessment. Documentation is the final step in a comprehensive pain assessment.

2
Pain Assessment

A rapid pain assessment includes:

- Type
- Severity
- Location
- Onset
- Duration
- History of previous pain

TERMS

- ☐ anxiety
- ☐ assess
- ☐ comprehensive pain assessment
- ☐ confidentiality
- ☐ confusion
- ☐ disclosure
- ☐ discomfort
- ☐ documentation
- ☐ duration
- ☐ fifth vital sign
- ☐ intensity
- ☐ location
- ☐ mental status
- ☐ onset
- ☐ open-ended questions
- ☐ pain scale
- ☐ physical assessment
- ☐ self efficacy
- ☐ severity
- ☐ therapeutic presence
- ☐ type
- ☐ vital signs

CASE STUDY

Mr. N., a 27-year-old chemical engineer, presents to the emergency room complaining of abdominal pain, nausea, vomiting and diarrhea for two days. He describes the pain as being most severe in the lower right quadrant and at the umbilicus. On physical exam, the nurse notes guarding behavior and rebound tenderness. Mr. N. reports he initially thought it was food poisoning, but no one else who ate sushi with him two evenings ago has been sick. Using open-ended questions, the nurse encourages Mr. N. to describe the duration and quality of his pain. She shows him a linear numeric pain scale and he describes the severity of his pain as "6 to 8." He explains that the pain interferes with his sleep. When asked, he states he has never experienced such severe pain: "8 out of 10." Self-prescribed Pepto-Bismol has not relieved the pain, nor has a heating pad.

 ## COMPREHENSIVE PAIN ASSESSMENT

Prior to designing or implementing an intervention for a client's symptom or problem, the nurse must be able to **assess** the problem. A **comprehensive pain assessment** is essential to identifying interventions appropriate for each specific client and each specific episode of pain. Assessing for pain includes collecting both subjective and objective data. Initial, rapid assessment of the client in pain should include identification of the **type**, **severity** (or **intensity**), **onset**, **duration**, **location**, and previous history of the pain. Both effective and ineffective self-care strategies should also be elicited. The pain experience should be described in the client's words. Some clients may avoid using the word pain and may actually deny pain as a problem, preferring to use a word such as "**discomfort**" instead. Acknowledgement of the client's personal description is essential to estab-

Complaints of pain should be described in the client's words; these descriptive words can offer insight into the type, severity, and cause of the pain.

Does the client mean pain when he says discomfort?

Assessment of the client in pain should include identification of the type, severity (or intensity), onset, duration, location, and previous history of the pain.

lishing effective communication, and this description should be adhered to in subsequent assessments.

Additional data in a comprehensive pain assessment includes identification of physiological signs and symptoms of pain, **vital signs**, a medical history, and assessment of psychosocial and cultural factors (**Table 2-1**). The American Pain Society has challenged all healthcare systems to regard pain as the **fifth vital sign**. Considering pain as a vital sign would ensure that pain is monitored on a regular basis and ideally would signal a need for further assessment and treatment.

 Frequently, clients do not seek medical care until their symptoms interfere with everyday life or are resistant to attempts at self-care.

Incomplete data collection, especially when related to healthcare provider biases or assumptions about pain, can lead to failure to offer useful interventions or cause further harm to the client. The client's pain sometimes impedes comprehensive assessment. Full assessment can be time-consuming; a variety of assessment and **documentation** strategies are useful in streamlining the task of assessing the client in pain.

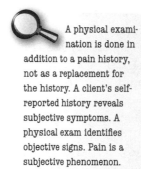 A physical examination is done in addition to a pain history, not as a replacement for the history. A client's self-reported history reveals subjective symptoms. A physical exam identifies objective signs. Pain is a subjective phenomenon.

Assessment Strategies

Assessment is a transpersonal relationship, a sharing exchange between caregiver and client. The client trades knowledge or information for high-quality nursing care. The caregiver would be unable to design a plan of care that is specific to the needs of the client without

Table 2-1 Rapid Pain Assessment

A rapid pain assessment includes:
- Type
- Severity
- Location
- Onset
- Duration
- History of previous pain

assessment information. In using the assessment to identify problems and past interventions, the healthcare professional provides the structure for the exchange. Several strategies are useful in structuring and streamlining the assessment process.

Pain is a subjective experience. The client's perspective is the most important source for assessment. Concentrating on the perspectives of others, such as spouse, family, or other healthcare providers, may result in barriers to pain relief.

Privacy

Privacy is fundamental to the assessment process. Much of the information revealed during assessment is of a personal nature, not easily shared under uncomfortable circumstances. A private, comfortable area should be available to conduct assessment activities. In addition to protecting the client and maintaining **confidentiality**, it is also a matter of health provider judgment whether to exclude the significant other from all or part of the assessment process. For many clients, the presence of a spouse

By denying pain, or lying about severity or intensity of pain, clients may choose to protect family members from knowing how bad the pain truly is.

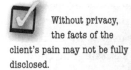

Without privacy, the facts of the client's pain may not be fully disclosed.

or parent is a comfort, but in other instances, the nature of the information shared is confidential. Clients may choose to protect family from knowledge of the severity of the pain. Methods of pain relief may also be confidential. Without privacy, the facts of the client's pain may not be fully disclosed. In another circumstance, the significant other may attempt to answer all assessment questions for the client. In this situation, only the significant other's perception of the client's pain is assessed. Pain is a subjective experience. Assessment should primarily include the client's perspective. Use of the significant other's input in addition to thorough client assessment may be useful.

Comfort

When a client is uncomfortable, assessment may be hindered. The environment in which an assessment is conducted should be clean, well lit, and relatively free of distractions. A chair may be more comfortable than an exam table for some clients. The temperature of the area should be warm enough for the client who is only partially clothed, or a blanket should be provided. Attempts should be made to minimize interruptions. When the nurse must respond to multiple requests or tasks during the assessment, important information may be missed. It is also important to maintain control of the interview, restricting the discussion primarily to the area of desired information. Many clients, especially the elderly or isolated clients, regard the assessment interview as an opportunity to visit or socialize. Assessment is essential to providing client care. Through minimizing distractions, interruptions, and extraneous information, the process will take less time and be more productive.

 Multiple interruptions during the assessment process may result in incomplete information and diminished trust in the caregiver-client relationship.

Structure the Assessment Interview

As in many client interactions, it is important to remember to ask **open-ended questions** during the pain assessment, allowing the client freedom to respond. This practice will enhance information shared and prevent caregiver biases from obscuring client data. Incorporating a framework into the assessment process assists in obtaining data and identifying missing elements. Two examples of assessment framework commonly used by nurses include head-to-toe assessment and functional health patterns. Choosing a framework should reflect the nurse's personal comfort and knowledge, as well as the structure of documentation required.

 The use of open ended questions in the assessment interview is one way to prevent caregiver bias and gives the client a voice in his pain management.

 Examples of open-ended questions:
- Tell me about your pain.
- Describe how you are feeling.
- What does it feel like?
- Tell me how this began.
- What other experiences have you had with pain?

Therapeutic Presence

While conducting a pain assessment, the provider utilizes **therapeutic presence**, projecting an air of caring concern. Clients will not share information with a professional whom they perceive to be uninterested

or distracted. Body language is one component of this presence. During the interview,
the provider should appear receptive with
professional dress and posture, and hands
still and visible. The provider should sit at
the same level as the client, avoiding a position of authority over the client. When culturally appropriate, the provider should also
maintain eye contact. The provider should
speak in a clear, calm tone, using language
and terms easily understood by the client and verifying the client's understanding of the questions asked.

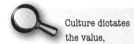

Culture dictates
the value,
meaning, and demonstra-
tion of pain. It may also
impede communication
about pain either from the
client's cultural perspective
or the heathcare profes-
sional's cultural biases.

BARRIERS TO ASSESSMENT

Physiological Barriers to Assessment

Just as an inadequate assessment is a barrier to pain management, there are many
barriers to the assessment process as well.
Pain is one of the primary barriers. Careful assessment for any signs of discomfort,
such as grimacing at rest or with movement,
is at least as important as verbal complaints
of pain. The client suffering from pain has a
shortened attention span and may not communicate clearly. The pain inhibits the client
from comprehending other stimuli. In such
an instance, the pain becomes an obstacle to
efforts for relief. The client's physical condition, in addition to pain, may impede con-
ducting a pain assessment. The client may be severely hard-of-hearing,
comatose, or have other factors inhibiting verbal communication.

Is there
congruence
between verbal and
nonverbal signs of pain?

Nonverbal
symptoms of
pain include grimacing at
rest or with movement,
guarding, crying, moaning,
changes in vital signs,
depression-like symptoms,
decrease in physical
activity.

Psychosocial Barriers to Assessment

The **mental status** of the client, which may or may not be pain-mediated,
can be another barrier to assessment. **Anxiety**, which often accompa-

nies pain, reduces comprehension, memory, and the ability to communicate. A client in pain may experience significant anxiety as a byproduct of or related to hospitalization, treatment, diagnostic procedures, role difficulties, or a variety of factors totally unrelated to his or her state of health. Acknowledging and addressing the state of anxiety and possible causes may be necessary prior to a pain assessment. If this is not possible, several steps can be taken to accommodate the anxious state. The provider should make an effort to speak slowly and clearly, frequently validating the client's understanding of questions and client responses. A quiet, nonthreatening environment should be maintained, and activities should be varied to accommodate the client's shortened attention span. For example, questions can be interjected while performing parts of the **physical assessment**. Severe anxiety may necessitate using an alternate history source, such as the client's family member or medical record.

Confusion is another problem that may interfere with assessment activities. It may be the result of a physiological condition such as hypoxia, blood loss, low blood pressure, hypoglycemia, electrolyte imbalances, medication ingestion, psychological disorders, or central nervous system disease. Other factors implicated in confusion include changes in diet and nutritional status, changes in environment and routine, trauma, and age. The elderly and very young are more apt to become confused when removed from a familiar environment, routine, and caregivers. Identifying the related factors to confusion and attempting correction when possible (such as administration of oxygen in a hypoxemic client) may allow for a more comprehensive pain assessment.

Time is a common barrier to comprehensive assessment, both because the client may not be physically present or available for prolonged periods and because of multiple demands placed on the provider's time. Organizational skills and realistic ordering of priorities may help resolve the problem of time constraints. Limited time should not impede an adequate assessment. Pain assessment is not a luxury: it is a requirement for provision of adequate care.

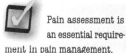 Pain assessment is an essential requirement in pain management.

 Confusion, resulting in shortened attention span, may interfere with assessment activities.

Language and culture are two other potential barriers to pain assessment. Culture dictates the value and meaning of the pain experience, as well as the conditions around **disclosure**. In some cultures, pain is experienced stoically—neither complained about nor even described. In other cultures, pain is expected and, in some instances, loudly vocalized. One example of this is childbirth during which, in certain cultures, the mother loudly proclaims her discomfort. It is part of the ritual of giving birth. Language, as a cultural barrier to assessment, is problematic when an appropriate interpreter is unavailable. It is important to note that many clients who speak English as a second language are much better able to communicate in their primary language during periods of intense stress or discomfort. Family members should not be used as interpreters, if at all possible, to maintain client confidentiality and to ensure factual information. Language may also inhibit the assessment process when the client or healthcare provider does not understand the other's use of medical jargon, street vernacular, or slang.

Often, family members seem to be more convenient or accessible, but are inappropriate as interpreters because of issues concerning client confidentiality.

The environment in which an assessment is conducted can provide multiple barriers to the process. Noise, frequent interruptions, a sense of lack of privacy, discomfort, and depersonalization can be part of the healthcare facility's environment. Depersonalization occurs when the client perceives that he or she is not valued or respected as a person and that what he or she is saying is not being listened to or used in planning his or her care. This may be a direct result of fear or distrust of the healthcare system or providers, or may be related to the attitude or actions of the healthcare provider. Minimizing the importance of a client's input, treating him or her like a child, or reducing his or her ability or opportunity to make realistic decisions concerning his care also contributes to a sense of depersonalization.

The immersion of a client in the sick role may also be responsible for depersonalization. The role of an ill individual often includes relinquishment of activities and responsibilities. However, it should also include efforts to return to a state of good health with a goal of participation in activities of daily living.

Hopelessness or powerlessness can have a major impact on the client's participation in the assessment process. If the client perceives that nothing can be done to relieve his or her pain or that he or she, personally, is

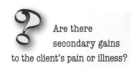

Are there secondary gains to the client's pain or illness?

unable to participate in productive activities to provide pain relief, participation in the pain assessment will be minimal. Listening to the client, assessing for flattened affect, reluctance to participate, or a history of conflict with healthcare providers will indicate clues to hopelessness or powerlessness.

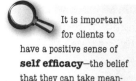

It is important for clients to have a positive sense of **self efficacy**—the belief that they can take meaningful action to impact their symptoms.

Finally, lack of access to a competent historian may inhibit pain assessment. There should be documentation as to who is providing the history. If the source is not the client, the perception of the pain experience is objective, not subjective.

CASE STUDY REVISITED

The nurse asks Mr. N. to describe his pain, to which he responds: "It is a sharp, throbbing, aching pain in my belly. Can't you give me something for it?" During physical assessment, and the time it takes for a CT scan, sonogram, and complete blood count to confirm a diagnosis of acute appendicitis, Mr. N. becomes more agitated and uncomfortable. As he is waiting for the surgeon to arrive, he suddenly reports feeling pain-free, stating: "I'm really better now. I think it was just gas. I'd like to go home!"

 ## PAIN HISTORY

The initial step in a comprehensive pain history is to interview the client, collecting a subjective history of the pain. Using the strategies discussed previously, the nurse asks open-ended questions about the type, location, severity, and nature of the pain. Listen carefully to the descriptors offered

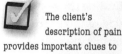

The client's description of pain provides important clues to the origin of that pain, guiding the nurse in appropriate interventions.

by the client. His description of the pain may indicate the source or type of pain. One excellent example is the burning, hot feeling described by the client suffering from herpetic shingles. The pain results from the inflammation of the nerve along which the herpes lesion is growing. Nerve pain, or neuroleptic pain, is commonly described using words like hot, burning, searing, or scalding. The competent historian responds to these clues when designing interventions. Neuroleptic pain does not commonly respond to narcotics, making them a poor choice for relief with this type of pain.

Location of the pain should be as specific as the client can describe. Avoid broad descriptive terms like "stomach ache." Determine where the pain originates and whether it radiates to other areas of the body. If pain is present in more than one area of the body, does the client relate the pains, or feel they are separate occurrences? Investigate what exacerbates or diminishes the pain. Identify activities that provide relief, such as change in position, eating, emptying the bladder. Identify measures the client has tried for pain relief and their effect.

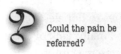 Could the pain be referred?

Determine how long the client has been in pain. Assess whether it is a recent occurrence or the intensification of a chronic condition. While assessing duration, ask about the consistency of the pain. Find out if it is constant and unremitting, or if it is intermittent in nature. If the pain is intermittent, ask if there is a cyclic quality, or if the pain recurs with some identified stimulus. Does the pain occur at certain times of the day or night? Does it cause the client to awake from sleep?

Intensity or severity of pain is assessed using a **pain scale**, allowing for rating of the pain. A variety of imaginative scales are available for use, and choice of scale is determined by the client's ability to communicate the intensity of the pain most accurately. A linear analogue or visual analogue (**Figure 2-1**) is considered the easiest for adults. This scale utilizes a line with qualifiers at one end, such as 0 (no pain), and 10 at the opposite end, indicating the worst pain one could ever imagine. Numeric scales will often utilize numbers from 0 to 10 at regular intervals (**Figure 2-2**). The client indicates how severe his or her pain is along the linear scale. The Acute

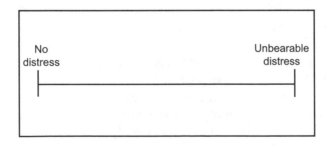

Figure 2-1 Visual analog scale (VAS).

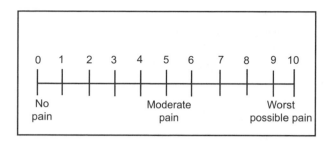

Figure 2-2 0 to 10 numerical pain intensity scale.

Pain Management Panel recommends standardizing linear and numerical scales along a 10 cm line. Standardized scales provide the opportunity for enhanced communication about the pain.

A descriptive scaling of pain is an alternative for assisting a client in his or her rating of the pain. Words are placed in order of severity (such as no pain, mild discomfort, painful, terribly painful, and unbearable pain). The provider reads the words to the client and asks him or her to choose the descriptor that best describes the severity of the pain. Numbers correspond with each descriptor, with 0 indicating no pain, 1 indicating mild pain, and so forth; the higher the number, the more severe the pain (**Figure 2-3**).

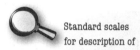

Standard scales for description of pain severity enhance communication, validate successive interventions, and provide more reliable evaluation of relief methods. Standard scales help us all to speak the same language about the pain. The use of these scales also aids in comparing pain from one instance to another or even one individual to another. This gives us a basis for research-based (evidence-based) practice.

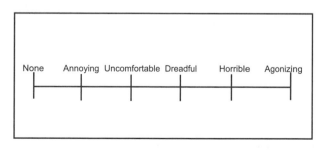

Figure 2-3 Simple descriptive pain distress scale.

A variety of other visual pain scales have been developed for use in assessment. Some include the use of color, either in discrete blocks or shading. These may be combined with descriptive words or numeric ranking (**Figure 2-4**). It is important to note that color may be interpreted differently by different cultures. Color may also be more expensive to duplicate when copying the scale for the use of other heath professionals. Line drawings or cartoons of simple facial expressions ranging from happy through grimacing are useful with children and nonverbal client populations (**Figure 2-5**).

Assess for symptoms that accompany the pain. These may include dizziness, photosensitivity, a sensation of light-headedness or feeling faint, nausea, diaphoresis, flushing or pallor, incontinence, weakness, loss of balance, redness, swelling, or warmth. Also assess for comorbidities: health problems that may change perception of pain or may impact the choice of interventions.

> Is the pain scale used appropriate for the client's developmental, visual, and verbal status, and is it being used consistently in the assessment process?

In assessing the nature of the pain, ask what impact it has on the client in terms of affecting mood, habits, and ability to participate in activities of daily living. Ask if the pain impacts sleep or rest, eating, mobility, or sexuality. Has the pain affected family dynamics or function in the workplace? Assess what the client suspects is the cause. Finally, ask the client to describe his or her history of pain: has he or she ever had pain like this before?

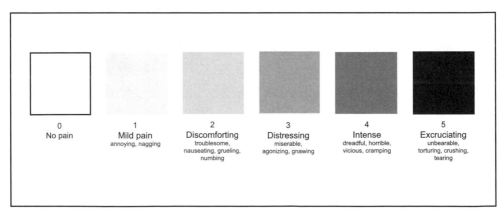

Figure 2-4 Pain assessment ruler (note: ruler is commonly in color. 0 = white; 1 = light blue; 2 = yellow; 3 = light orange; 4 = dark orange; 5 = red).

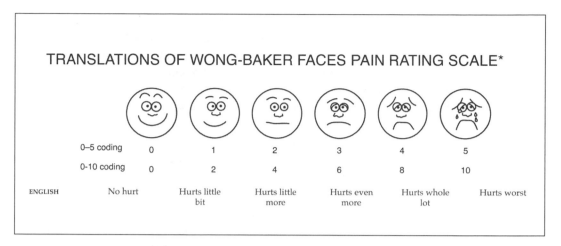

TRANSLATIONS OF WONG-BAKER FACES PAIN RATING SCALE*

0–5 coding	0	1	2	3	4	5
0-10 coding	0	2	4	6	8	10
ENGLISH	No hurt	Hurts little bit	Hurts little more	Hurts even more	Hurts whole lot	Hurts worst

Figure 2-5 Wong-Baker FACES pain rating scale. From Hockenberry MJ, Wilson D, Winkelstein ML: *Wong's Essentials of Pediatric Nursing*, ed. 7, St. Louis, 2005, p. 1259. Used with permission. Copyright, Mosby.

What relieved the pain? What are his or her other experiences with pain and pain relief, especially medications? Identify allergies or sensitivities to medications and current use of prescribed and unprescribed medications.

At the conclusion of a thorough pain history, the healthcare provider verifies information obtained with the client to avoid misunderstandings or incomplete data.

 Neglecting to verify information gathered during assessment can result in inappropriate or useless interventions to manage the pain.

 PHYSICAL ASSESSMENT

The physical assessment for pain involves identification of objective signs of pain. Although pain is primarily subjective, objective manifestations can be of value, especially when evaluating interventions for relief. It is not the goal of the pain assessment to diagnose the cause of pain. A rapid head-to-toe assessment can identify contributing factors as well as barriers to assessment. Vital signs may indicate a painful state, usually with an increase in heart rate, respirations, and an elevation in blood pressure. However, in some clients, blood pressure may decrease with severe pain.

State of consciousness and affect may vary with severe pain. Agitation is often associated with acute pain, while a flattened affect of withdrawal may be associated with chronic pain. Physical assessment of the painful area includes evaluation for redness, swelling, heat or cold, masses, and a functional assessment. Functional assessment includes sensation and movement of an affected extremity, bowel sounds in a painful abdomen, or heart and breath sounds in the case of chest pain. Physical assessment progresses from inspection through auscultation, then percussion (when these are indicated) to palpation. Percussion and palpation may exacerbate the client's pain. The client is asked to demonstrate positions or movements that increase or relieve the pain. Throughout the physical assessment, privacy and comfort are provided.

CASE STUDY REVISITED

The relief from pain indicates, at this point, that Mr. N.'s appendix has probably ruptured; surgery is now an emergency procedure, necessary to prevent further complications. Finishing a pain history, the nurse ascertains that Mr. N. has been treated for severe pain with morphine sulfate after breaking his leg. He reports that, at that time, symptoms including urinary retention and severe itching were associated with morphine use.

 Vital signs change with the presence of pain: increase in heart rate, respirations, and an elevation or decrease in blood pressure.

 Is the client describing changes in sensation and movement, bowel activity, or palpitations or shortness of breath?

 ## DOCUMENTING PAIN ASSESSMENT

Documentation is the final step in a comprehensive pain assessment. It is an important step in communication among members of the healthcare team so that the information can be used in planning interventions for pain relief, as well as diagnosing the cause of the pain. Excellent documentation of pain assessment allows the practitioner to evaluate relief measures as well as improvement or decline in the client's condition. An initial pain assessment may be quite lengthy. It can be documented as a narrative note; however, a common framework should be used. It may consist of the assessment framework, such as the head-to-toe method or an independent framework incorporating all aspects of the assessment process. It must include type, severity (or intensity), onset, duration, location, and history of previous pain.

Flow sheets have been developed for pain assessment, incorporating multiple assessments as well as space to document intervention and evaluation. The severity may be documented as a number value if using a standard scale, or a linear or visual analog may be displayed and marked at each pain assessment. Some facilities include an anatomical drawing, front and back, so that the location of the pain can be drawn or indicated (**Figure 2-6**). Medications used for pain control should be documented, including the dose, route, duration of use, side effects experienced, and the client's view of efficacy. Interventions that are not effective should be discarded.

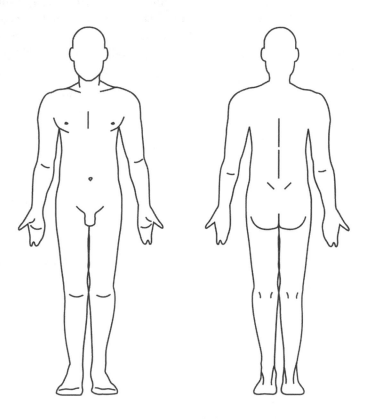

Figure 2-6 Drawings used to determine areas of pain and radiation.

Pain is not static; it may change often, due to multiple factors. For this reason, pain assessments should be done frequently, on a regular basis, and documented clearly and completely. Healthcare providers should not wait for a client complaint to institute further assessment. It is essential to remember that the client is the very best indicator of pain; pain is what the client describes it to be.

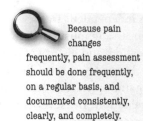 Because pain changes frequently, pain assessment should be done frequently, on a regular basis, and documented consistently, clearly, and completely.

CASE STUDY RESOLVED

After completing Mr. N.'s assessment, the nurse documents her findings in the chart, as well as sharing information about adverse effects of morphine with the surgeon. The plan is made to treat Mr. N.'s postoperative pain using subcutaneous Demerol, instead of morphine. His pain remains well controlled, and he is discharged from the hospital on an oral opioid and antibiotic on the third postoperative day.

CHAPTER 2 · REVIEW QUESTIONS

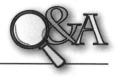

1. The most essential step to providing pain management for an individual client is a:
    A. Comprehensive pain assessment
    B. Comprehensive health history
    C. Written plan of care
    D. Familiarity with prescription medications often used for pain control

2. A comprehensive pain assessment includes information concerning:
    A. Type of pain
    B. Duration of pain
    C. Medication history
    D. All of the above

3. Which of the following are potential barriers to pain assessment?
    A. Language and culture
    B. Diet and exercise
    C. Site and duration of pain
    D. Client education

4. The following scale is appropriate to measure pain in the 3-year-old child:
    A. Linear scale marked 1 through 10
    B. A "faces of pain" scale illustrating happy through crying
    C. A linear scale with printed words describing pain
    D. A verbal scale with words describing the pain

5. During a physical assessment for pain, it is important for the nurse to consider that:
    A. Chronic pain and acute pain are frequently expressed in the same manner
    B. Pain is only a subjective phenomenon
    C. There is a characteristic shift in vital signs for all clients in pain
    D. Chronic pain can be expressed very differently from acute pain

6. Functional assessment of the client with pain should include:
   A. The client's ability to complete activities of daily living
   B. The client's willingness to use prescribed remedies
   C. Extended social support for the client
   D. Function of major organ systems

7. Pain assessment should be done:
   A. Only once
   B. Once each shift or visit
   C. By one single caregiver
   D. Repeatedly to assist with managing fluctuations or changes in the client's pain

ANSWERS AND RATIONALES

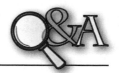

1. **A.** This assessment includes both subjective and objective data.

2. **D.** All are important in formulating a plan of care for the client experiencing pain.

3. **A.** Culture and/or language may affect how pain is expressed.

4. **B.** is most appropriate, allowing the child to communicate using visual cues. Numbers and words are less appropriate because of developmental level and the potential for developmental regression during pain or illness.

5. **D.** Individuals with chronic pain may appear very different from those with acute pain.

6. **A.** Ability to participate in activities of daily living, including self-care and life roles, is part of the functional assessment.

7. **D.** Continual assessment improves pain management.

REFERENCES

Acute Pain Management Clinical Practice Guideline Panel. (1992). *Acute pain management: operative or medical procedures and trauma. AHCPR Pub No. 92-0032.* Rockville, MD: Agency for Health Care Policy and Research, U.S. Department of Health and Human Services, Public Health Service.

Mayer, D. D., Torma, L., Byock, I., & Norris, K. (2001). Speaking the language of pain. *Am J Nurs*, *101*(2), 44–50.

McCaffery M., & Pasero, C. (1999). *Pain: clinical manual* (2nd ed.). St. Louis, MO: Mosby;.

Platt, A. F., & Byrnes, J. F. (2006). Pain assessment tools: guide for healthcare professionals. *Patient Care for the Nurse Practitioner.* Available at: http://patientcarenp.com. Accessed May 2007.

Torma, L. A. Pain as the fifth vital sign task force. Missoula Demonstration Project: The Quality of Life's End. Available at: http://www.missoulademonstration.org/fifth_vital_sign_tf.shtml. Accessed September 21, 2007.

RELATED WEBSITES

The Agency for Healthcare Research and Quality: www.ahrq.gov

The American Academy of Pain Management: www.aapainmanage.org

The American Academy of Pain Medicine: www.painmed.org

The American Chronic Pain Association: www.theacpa.org

The American Pain Foundation: www.painfoundation.org

The American Pain Society: www.ampainsoc.org

The American Society of Pain Management Nurses: www.aspmn.org

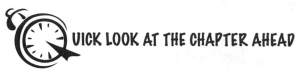
Once effective assessment of pain is complete, pain management strategies must be identified to promote optimal pain relief. Some ways to manage the client's pain may be pharmacological, including analgesics, opioids, and anesthetics. Other options may be physiological, including methods of transcutaneous stimulation, postural changes, or use of acupuncture or acupressure points. Finally, behavioral measures including education, relaxation, guided imagery, or other client choices can be incorporated into the plan. The plan of care may include traditional medical approaches as well as nontraditional, cultural, or religious variables, which may be identified either by the client or caregiver. When designing the plan of care, it is important to include both traditional and nontraditional interventions for optimal relief, rather than take an all-or-none approach. One single intervention rarely provides complete relief for the client. This chapter will provide a review of many of the pain management strategies available, but research continually uncovers new strategies as well as innovative and different ways to utilize old ones.

3

Interventions for Pain

TERMS
- ☐ acupressure
- ☐ acupuncture
- ☐ adjuvant medications
- ☐ aromatherapy
- ☐ around-the-clock dosage schedules
- ☐ biofeedback
- ☐ cultural alternatives
- ☐ distraction
- ☐ equianalgesic
- ☐ guided imagery
- ☐ massage
- ☐ nonopioid analgesics
- ☐ nonsteroidal anti-inflammatory drugs (NSAIDs)
- ☐ opioids
- ☐ over-the-counter medication
- ☐ potentiators
- ☐ prescription medication
- ☐ PRN
- ☐ therapeutic touch
- ☐ touch
- ☐ transcutaneous electric nerve stimulation (TENS)

CASE STUDY

Mrs. L., a 48-year-old woman who is active and in excellent health, has torn her anterior cruciate ligament (ACL) while waterskiing. She now complains of severe pain, which interferes with her usually very active lifestyle. She has used ibuprofen for pain relief with poor success. She states that she has been unable to ride her bike, that kneeling to do her gardening has become impossible, and that even walking has become painful.

On physical examination, her knee is swollen, red, and warm to touch. Because Mrs. L. is in good health and prefers her previous level of activity, ACL repair is planned.

 ## MEDICATION FOR PAIN MANAGEMENT

Medication is a commonly used and well-received intervention for pain management. It is used with or without the participation of a healthcare provider. The client or client's family may choose an **over-the-counter medication** perceived as appropriate to the client's symptoms or may choose to use a **prescription medication** either left over from a previous experience with pain or belonging to someone other than the client. When the client chooses to contact the health-care provider for treatment of pain, he or she often expects medication as an intervention.

A wide variety of medications are available for pain management. They include commonly used "pain" medications as well as adjuvant medicines, which moderate factors that can cause or aggravate pain or mediate the activity of the primary medication. Medications that treat the cause of the pain are also instrumental in relieving pain. Medication for specific painful conditions such as angina or neuroleptic pain can be used. Rarely is a single medication successful in alleviating pain unless it is used to treat pain with a very specific causative factor or the pain is quite mild.

 Despite the fact that medication is the primary expectation when a client seeks out a healthcare provider for pain management, one single intervention rarely provides complete relief for the client.

 The "five rights" for medication administration safety are:
1. The right drug
2. The right dose
3. The right time
4. The right route
5. The right client

Nonsteroidal Anti-inflammatory Drugs (NSAIDs)

Pain is usually classified as mild, moderate, or severe. Severity of pain, along with type and location, are parameters used in initially choosing a medication protocol. Common pain medications include **nonopioid analgesics** and **opioids** (narcotics). Nonopioids include acetaminophen, salicylates like aspirin, and **nonsteroidal anti-inflammatory drugs (NSAIDs)** including ibuprofen. These medications, some of which also have antipyretic or anti-inflammatory properties, are chosen to treat mild to moderate pain. With the advent of availability of over-the-counter NSAIDs several years ago (e.g., Motrin, Advil), all three of these types of medications are available to clients for self-treatment of mild to moderate pain.

Dose Schedules

One drawback in the use of these medications is dosage scheduling. They may be prescribed by healthcare professionals or used by clients on an as needed (**PRN**) basis, not taken until pain is evident or until discomfort is becoming worse. It becomes more of a challenge to alleviate present pain than to prevent recurrence of pain. For this reason, **around-the-clock dosage schedules** may be more effective for optimal pain relief.

 Prevention of pain or of increased severity of pain is a more desirable outcome than treating pain that has already begun or is increasing in severity.

Therefore, around-the-clock dosing is significantly more effective for optimal pain relief.

Side Effects and Toxicity

Nonopioids are limited in that they have a ceiling or maximum safe dose beyond which significant toxicity can occur, presenting danger to the client. Each drug has its own specific ceiling and cluster of side effects, which should be known and readily recognized by the healthcare provider who is prescribing their use (**Table 3-1**). Most medications in these classes are available primarily in oral dose form; however, several are available in suppository form. Several rarely used NSAIDs are available for parenteral administration.

Acetaminophen, aspirin, and NSAIDs are relatively inexpensive, readily available, and do not cause central nervous system (CNS)-related side effects such as bowel or bladder problems, sedation, or respiratory depression. NSAIDs, however, can cause gastrointestinal bleeding because they block prostaglandin synthesis and can interfere with the mucosal barrier of the gastrointestinal tract.

Table 3-1 Dosing Data for Oral NSAIDs

Drug	Usual Adult Dose	Usual Pediatric Dose	Comments
Acetaminophen	650–975 mg q 4 hrs	10–15 mg/kg q 4 hrs	Lacks the peripheral anti-inflammatory activity of other NSAIDs
Aspirin	650–975 mg q 4 hrs	10–15 mg/kg q 4 hrs	Standard against which other NSAIDs are compared; inhibits platelet aggregation; may cause postop bleeding
Choline magnesium trisalicylate (Trilisate)	1000–1500 mg BID	25 mg/kg BID	May have minimal antiplatelet activity; also available as oral liquid
Diflunisal (Dolobid)	1000 mg initial dose followed by 500 mg q 12 hrs		
Etodolac (Lodine)	200–400 mg q 6–8 hrs		
Fenoprofen (Nalfon)	200 mg q 4–6 hrs calcium		
Ibuprofen (Motrin, etc)	400 mg q 4–6 hrs	10 mg/kg q 6–8 hrs	Many brand names and generic available; also as oral suspension
Ketoprofen (Orudis)	25–75 mg q 6–8 hrs		
Magnesium salicylate	650 mg q 4 hrs		Many brands and generic forms available

Note: From Acute Pain Management Guideline Panel. (1992). *Acute Pain Management: Operative or Medical Procedures and Trauma. Clinical Practice Guideline. AHCPR Pub No. 92-0032.* Rockville, Md: Agency for Health Care Policy and Research, Public Health Service, U.S. Department of Health and Human Service.

Because renal function depends on prostaglandins, NSAIDS should also be used cautiously in individuals with impaired renal function. Each year there are approximately 107,000 hospitalizations with more

than 16,500 deaths related to side effects of
NSAIDs. Individuals at risk for gastrointestinal side effects of NSAIDs may be given cy-
clooxygenase isoenzyme (COX-2) inhibitors
for their analgesic effect. COX-2 inhibitors
have a better safety profile than NSAIDs because of their sparing effect on platelet aggregation and on the gastrointestinal tract.
Although these COX-2 inhibitors have decreased risk for gastrointestinal bleeding,
they too are contraindicated in some client
populations. Caution should be taken when considering COX-2 inhibiters
for clients who have had allergic reactions to sulfonamides or in clients
who have experienced asthma, urticaria, or allergic reactions after taking
aspirin or other NSAIDs.

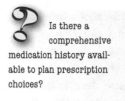

Is there a
comprehensive
medication history avail-
able to plan prescription
choices?

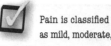

Pain is classified
as mild, moderate,
or severe.

Opioids

When pain is moderate to severe, or NSAID or COX-2 inhibitor therapy
has failed, the addition of an opioid to the treatment plan is indicated.
However, it is important to consider if the
failure is related to PRN dosing. Prior to
adding an opioid, review the NSAIDs dosage schedule. If PRN dosing was used, it may
be possible to have success with NSAIDs
administered around-the-clock.

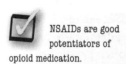

NSAIDs are good
potentiators of
opioid medication.

Opioids work by binding with opioid receptor sites in the central and
peripheral nervous systems. Using NSAIDs in combination with opioids
usually results in effective pain management with smaller necessary doses
of opioids, thereby reducing the risk of CNS side effects associated with
opioid use. In addition to CNS side effects, opioids are associated with
physical tolerance and psychological dependence. Physical tolerance is
unusual in the client with pain using opioids for a short period.

Codeine, oxycodone, morphine, meperidine (Demerol®) and hydrocodone are all opioids commonly used in pain management. Oral forms
of codeine, oxycodone, and hydrocodone are often used to treat moderate
pain in combination with acetaminophen. Oxycodone and hydrocodone
are not available in parenteral formulations, so codeine may be chosen
for those clients who cannot tolerate oral medication. Clients often report nausea, vomiting, sedation, and feelings of "disconnectedness" with

these medications. If one of these medications causes unpleasant side effects such as nausea, the client may be able to tolerate one of the other choices. Codeine and the codeine derivatives are frequently prescribed as pain therapy following outpatient invasive procedures, including diagnostics and dental surgery. They are inexpensive and come in combination tablet form with NSAIDs. It is important to be aware of the ceiling dose of the combined NSAID when titrating medication dosages upward for pain relief.

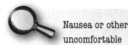 Nausea or other uncomfortable symptoms are not necessarily cause for discontinuing or changing a medication for pain. If acceptable pain management is possible, try treating the symptom rather than changing medications.

Morphine sulfate and hydromorphone (Dilaudid®) are more commonly used for severe pain or after procedures when it is expected that severe pain will occur, such as major surgery. These medications are often administered parenterally, but addition of an NSAID when the client can tolerate oral medication may increase comfort and decrease the need for opioids.

Meperidine is another medication used after procedures, but it is not recommended in elders or in clients with renal dysfunction. If meperidine is given parenterally, it should only be used for 48 hours because of the risk of meperidine toxicity. When meperidine is prescribed, doses should be adequate to provide good pain relief and given frequently enough. It is often prescribed in inadequate doses with no consideration for its very short serum half-life.

 Never use meperidine in patients with renal dysfunction, or patients at high risk for renal dysfunction, such as diabetics.

Morphine sulfate is the "gold standard" for opioid pain relief. It is against this standard that dosing and efficacy are measured and equianalgesic tables are constructed. It is available in oral, parenteral, and rectal preparations, as well as in immediate-release and extended-release oral forms. Clients using morphine may experience nausea and vomiting, which usually resolves within 24 hours of the first dose and is responsive to conventional antiemetic therapy. Itching is another unpleasant side effect described by a small percentage of clients who use morphine. Inability to provide comfort from these side effects requires consideration of a different opioid for pain relief.

In addition to sedation and respiratory depression, opioids can cause constipation, which can have a significantly negative impact on quality of life. Baseline bowel assessment should be done, with continued assessment for regular bowel activity during opioid use. Addition of extra fluids and extra fiber to the diet or a bulk laxative with adequate fluid intake should be instituted when the client can tolerate it.

Efficacy of opioid use depends on assessment or evaluation for pain relief, as well as the presence of medication side effects. Poor relief in the absence of side effects indicates the need for increased doses of the opioid. Other medications that enhance the activity of the opioid or reduce factors that cause or exacerbate pain should also be considered for use. These are called **adjuvant medications**—drugs used in addition to the already prescribed therapy. Use of adjuvant medications does not preclude continuing to use NSAIDs previously incorporated into the opioid regimen.

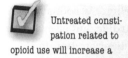

Untreated constipation related to opioid use will increase a client's level of discomfort.

Potentiators of opioids include benzodiazepines and phenothiazines. Anti-anxiety medications such as diazepam (Valium®) or lorazepam (Ativan®) promote relaxation, may reduce muscular tension, and reduce anxiety. Lorazepam and antihistamines also act as antiemetics, reducing nausea and vomiting. Diphenhydramine (Benadryl®), a common antihistamine, when used with morphine can help to relieve nausea and itching. Steroids reduce inflammation. It is important to consider undesirable side effects, such as increased sedation, which may be enhanced by the adjuvant medications.

Finally, certain medications are specific to certain pain syndromes. Neuroleptic or nerve pain is poorly relieved with traditional doses of opioids, and the pain is often too severe to respond solely to anti-inflammatory therapy. Phantom pain following amputation or pain from nerve compression by tumor or fracture are two good examples of this type of pain. Tricyclic antidepressants and anticonvulsant medications are very useful in relieving this type of pain. However, it has been demonstrated that larger-than-usual doses of opioids, particularly morphine, effectively relieve this type of pain. In place of large doses of morphine, some practitioners consider the use of methadone, which is highly effective but has greater risk of multiple side effects.

Methadone has been used in treatment of opioid addiction but is currently being used in treatment of severe pain. It is a drug that, with repeated dosing, has high affinity for the mu receptors and demonstrates greater efficacy than other opioid drugs. For this reason, it is a very good choice for treating pain, such as neuroleptic pain, at lower doses than morphine. Severe toxicities may not become evident until several days of methadone therapy, so great care should be taken when starting methadone as medication for pain management.

Cardiac anginal pain, which occurs as the result of inadequate oxygen to the myocardium, responds to morphine partly because the sedating effect reduces cardiac metabolism, simultaneously reducing the oxygen deficit. Vasodilators are successfully used to relieve anginal pain, both cardiac and elsewhere in the body, by increasing circulation and oxygen delivery to the affected area. Local anesthetic agents are used topically or subcutaneously for local pain control.

Routes of Administration

Choice and administration of medications include considering the "five rights" in client-focused safety: the right drug, the right dose, the right time, the right route, and the right client. Choosing an appropriate route for medication administration takes into consideration many factors. Oral

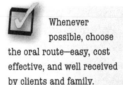 Whenever possible, choose the oral route—easy, cost effective, and well received by clients and family.

medication is commonly the easiest and most cost-effective route of choice. It is appropriate when the client can safely swallow and tolerate oral intake.

When oral administration is not an option, relatively less invasive routes include sublingual, rectal, and transcutaneous. Choices among these routes are dictated by the availability of medication for that particular route, as well as client-specific issues.

Injectable administration is a relatively more invasive or traumatic choice. Clients may have fears or preconceptions about receiving injections. There is a small chance of infection, especially with poor technique. Although small, the risk for infection is greater than with previously described administration choices. Subcutaneous injection allows for delivery and absorption of small volumes of fluid; intramuscular injection will accommodate larger volumes, but

 Clients and families can be taught to administer subcutaneous injections, but only if they are willing.

still no more than 2.5 cc. Absorption and delivery of medication to central circulation is slower and less reliable with subcutaneous injection. Poor peripheral circulation and loss of subcutaneous tissue further decrease the efficacy of medication delivery with subcutaneous injection.

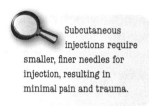

Subcutaneous injections require smaller, finer needles for injection, resulting in minimal pain and trauma.

Intramuscular injection results in quicker absorption, but reliability is dependent on muscle mass, activity, and peripheral circulation. Increased muscular activity or elevated body temperature can result in faster movement of the medication into central circulation. This can be particularly problematic with pain medication, as the drugs are moved away from the muscular storage and more rapidly metabolized, leaving the patient without effective pain management.

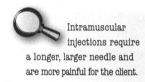

Intramuscular injections require a longer, larger needle and are more painful for the client.

Intravenous injection of medication allows for larger volumes of fluid as well as extremely rapid delivery. Medication administered intravenously has a shorter half-life within the body because it is more rapidly delivered to the liver and kidneys for clearance from the body. Intravenous infusion of opioids is potentially more dangerous because of the risk of overdose when the entire dose is delivered very rapidly. The antidote naloxone (Narcan®) should be readily available to completely block opioid action in case of accidental overdose when the intravenous route is used.

 Professional assistance is necessary for clients and families to manage intravenous administration outside of the hospital.

Intravenous administration of opioids is the route of choice when a patient-controlled analgesia (PCA) pump is used in the plan of care. The PCA pump allows the client to use a device to demand a computer-driven pump inject a predetermined dose of medication into an intravenous (IV) line. Maximum dose over a determined time frame is programmed into the pump computer, preventing the client from receiving any more medication than has been ordered. It is a safe and effective way of promoting client involvement in pain management, allowing client control over the medication. This alternative is more comfortable for clients than repeated, intermittent injections and is cost-effective, reducing nursing time spent with multiple intermittent administrations. Sophisticated pump computers allow the healthcare provider to track how frequently medication is requested by the client and whether a dose was delivered or not.

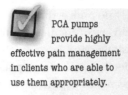 PCA pumps provide highly effective pain management in clients who are able to use them appropriately.

 PCA pump administration is impossible without appropriate and timely education for the client.

The client who can use a PCA pump must be motivated to use the equipment, able to learn how to use it, available for client education, and a candidate for IV administration of an opioid. Side effects of the opioid can certainly occur with use of a PCA pump. Oversedation is rare, because as the client becomes more sedated, requests for medication become less frequent. Other side effects such as nausea, itching, and confusion should be addressed immediately using conventional interventions or a change in medication. PCA pumps can be programmed to deliver a bolus of medication as requested, simulating a PRN dose schedule; or a basal rate of medication can be programmed for continuous infusion, with smaller boluses available for breakthrough pain or to increase activity tolerance, as requested by the client.

 ## EQUIANALGESIC PAIN MANAGEMENT

One of the most common errors made when changing pain management medication is undermedication, resulting in poor pain relief. When pain management is effective, but it is necessary to change either medication or route, an **equianalgesic** chart should be consulted so that the client will not be over- or undermedicated using the new route or medication.

 Always consider principles of equianalgesics when changing pain medication!

An excellent example of the need for a change, despite successful pain relief, is a situation in which a surgical client who has been maintained comfortably on the PCA pump is changed to oral (PO) medication in preparation for discharge home. It is vital to keep this client comfortable, enable increased mobility, and return the client to baseline activities of daily living. By identifying the amount of medication the client is currently receiving, a comparable amount of the new medication can be ordered. Even a change in route only requires reference to the equianalgesic table.

The table uses morphine as the standard, and comparable amounts of other medications and their routes are listed. The chart provides a guideline for initial dosing when making a change in drug and/or route (**Table 3-2**). For example, a client receiving morphine sulfate 3 mg IV every 3 hours for adequate pain control will be changed to Percocet® (oxycodone 5 mg and acetaminophen 325 mg) in preparation for discharge home. He has used Percocet with good effect in the past. Referring to the equianalgesic chart, the healthcare provider will order two Percocet tablets (oxycodone 10 mg and acetaminophen 650 mg) to be taken every 4 hours. It is essential to evaluate the client's pain relief on this new medication, with revisions made to the plan before discharge home.

CASE STUDY REVISITED

Upon return at 6:00 PM to the postoperative floor after uncomplicated ACL repair, Mrs. L. has morphine sulfate 2 to 3 mg SC q 2–3 hours PRN ordered for pain. She complains of moderate to severe pain throughout the evening, describing it as 7 on a scale of 1 to 10. She requests medication every 2 hours. She also complains of severe nausea. Her primary nurse realizes that it will be a long, uncomfortable night unless some changes are made in the plan of care.

A conversation with the surgeon results in new medication orders: meperidine (Demerol) 50 mg with hydroxyzine hydrochloride (Vistaril) 50 mg IM q 4 hours around-the-clock for pain. The nurse believes that this client would have been a good candidate for a PCA pump, but she has had no training to use one and is now too uncomfortable. She gives Mrs. L. her first shot of Demerol and Vistaril, explaining that the Vistaril not only makes the Demerol more effective but will help decrease the nausea. Mrs. L. reports feeling much more comfortable within the space of 1 hour.

The nurse also does some simple relaxation exercises with her, primarily controlled breathing and progressive muscle relaxation, and helps her

Table 3-2 Dose Equivalents for Opioid Analgesics in Opioid-Naive Clients > 50 kg Body Weight*

Drug	Approximate Equianalgesic Dose		Usual Starting Dose for Moderate to Severe Pain	
	Oral	*Parenteral*	*Oral*	*Parenteral*
Opioid Agonist** Morphine	30 mg q 3–4 hrs (repeat around-the-clock dosing) 60 mg q 3–4 hrs (single or intermittent dosing)	10 mg q 3–4 hrs	30 mg q 3–4 hrs	10 mg q 3–4 hrs
Morphine, controlled release (MS Contin, OraMorph)	90–120 mg q 12 hrs	N/A	90–120 mg q 12 hrs	N/A
Hydromorphone (Dilaudid)	7.5 mg q 3–4 hrs	1.5 mg q 3–4 hrs	6 mg q 3–4 hrs	1.5 mg q 3–4 hrs
Levorphanol (Levo-Dromoran)	4 mg q 6–8 hrs	2 mg q 6–8 hrs	4 mg q 6–8 hrs	2 mg q 6–8 hrs
Meperidine (Demerol)	300 mg q 2–3 hrs	100 mg q 3 hrs	N/R	100 mg q 3 hrs
Methadone (Dolophine, etc)	20 mg q 6–8 hrs	10 mg q 6–8 hrs	20 mg q 6–8 hrs	10 mg q 6–8 hrs
Oxymorphone (Numorphan)	N/A	1 mg q 3–4 hrs	N/A	1 mg q 3–4 hrs
Combination Opioid/NSAID Preparations+				
Codeine (with aspirin or acetaminophen)	180–200 mg q 3–4 hrs	130 mg q 3–4 hrs	60 mg q 3–4 hrs	60 mg q 2 hrs (IM/SC)
Hydrocodone (in Lorcet, Lortab, Vicodin, etc)	30 mg q 3–4 hrs	N/A	10 mg q 3–4 hrs	N/A
Oxycodone (Roxicodone, also in Percocet, Percodan, Tylox, etc)	30 mg q 3–4 hrs	N/A	10 mg q 3–4 hrs	N/A

*Caution: Recommended doses do not apply for adults with body weight < 50 kg.

**Caution: Recommended doses do not apply to clients with renal or hepatic insufficiency or other conditions affecting drug metabolism and kinetics.

+Caution: For these drugs, rectal administration is an alternate route for patients unable to take oral medications.

Note: From Acute Pain Management Guideline Panel. (1992). *Acute Pain Management: Operative or Medical Procedures and Trauma. Clinical Practice Guideline.* AHCPR Pub No. 92-0032. Rockville, Md: Agency for Health Care Policy and Research, Public Health Service, U.S. Department of Health and Human Service.

to change her position in bed. By 10:30 PM, Mrs. L. is sleeping, but the night nurse will be careful to continue to administer the IM pain medication even if the client is asleep, to prevent the recurrence of severe pain.

 # PHYSICAL STRATEGIES TO MANAGE PAIN

Manipulation and change in the client's physical status present another variety of pain control techniques. These are useful as adjuvant therapies in moderate to severe pain or may even be used alone when pain is mild or medication is poorly tolerated. Some of these strategies may be performed independently by the client, while others may require the assistance of another individual.

Touch

Touch is a simple strategy used in caring for the client in pain. Touch can provide reassurance, a sense of contact and involvement, and may facilitate relaxation. Muscular tension can be a causative factor for some types of pain or may be a contributing factor in others. Promoting reduced tension can assist with pain relief. Other types of cutaneous or transcutaneous stimulation can also be used in pain relief. Gentle cutaneous stimulation, either at the site of pain or at another site on the body, can have the effect of confounding the gate control for pain stimulus, short circuiting the system and reducing the perceived painful sensations. This light, rhythmic stroking with only a feather-light touch is called *effleurage*. It is often taught to pregnant women for use in labor pain management. It can be performed by a caregiver or by the client him- or herself.

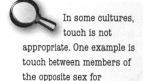
In some cultures, touch is not appropriate. One example is touch between members of the opposite sex for Orthodox Jews.

Massage

Massage is another form of touch that can be gentle or more vigorous. Gentle massage, in which stroking is rhythmic but not as light as effleurage, can reduce pain gate sensations or help to promote muscle relaxation. Deep massage, usually done by a healthcare provider or massage therapist, promotes relaxation and a sense of well-being but should

be used only in specific situations. Clients
with bleeding dyscrasias or who are at risk
for clot or thrombus formation are not candidates for massage. These clients are at risk
for bleeding, bruising, or embolization with

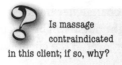

Is massage
contraindicated
in this client; if so, why?

massage. One good example is a client with leg pain as the result of a
deep vein thrombosis. Massage is especially beneficial for the client with
chronic pain. Reflexology is an ancient form of natural healing that uses
massage at reflex points on the feet. Specific points refer to specific body
areas and will promote relief from pain and healing in that area.

Heat or Cold Therapy

Application of heat or cold therapy is another form of cutaneous or transcutaneous stimulation that may promote pain relief. Application of cold
to the painful area results in slight numbing. The sensation of cold is
sent as a message to the central nervous system, short-circuiting the gate
control mechanism for pain. Decrease in local body temperature results
in slight vasoconstriction of the area, reducing local circulation as well
as limiting the amount of extracellular fluid leaking into the area. Limiting extracellular fluid reduces or prevents swelling. Swelling, through
increased local pressure, may increase or even be a cause of pain. It is
important when using application of cold to relieve pain to protect the
skin. Ice should not be applied directly; instead, it should be wrapped in
a towel or cloth. Cold should be applied intermittently. A good rule is 20
minutes on, 20 minutes off. Continuous application of cold could result
in tissue damage as the result of continued vasoconstriction.

 Continuous application of cold can damage tissue.

Use of heat in pain relief is another common choice. Warmth promotes muscular relaxation and a sense of comfort. As previously noted,
decreasing muscular tension may reduce pain sensations. Vasodilatation
occurs locally in the area where heat is applied. This increases circulation, enhancing the removal of cellular debris, toxins, and extracellular
fluid from the area of tissue injury. Although heat is not useful in preventing swelling, it is a great aid in reducing swelling that has already
occurred. Reduction in swelling may enhance comfort.

As with the application of cold, care should be taken to protect the
skin where heat is applied. The older client, or one with neuropathy, is at

risk for burns when heat injury is not noticed. Clients with mental status changes or who are sedated should not use heat for pain relief without supervision, as injury may result. Continuous application of heat is contraindicated for a variety of reasons. The same 20 on, 20 off rule used when applying cold is also a good idea for heat application. Temperature of any heating device should be frequently checked to prevent burns. Finally, heat should never be applied to an area where arterial vascular insufficiency is suspected. In this instance, metabolism and oxygen need are increased, putting the client in danger of injury from oxygen deficit.

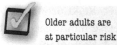 Older adults are at particular risk for injuries from heat therapy due to decreased subcutaneous tissue, poor peripheral circulation, and peripheral neuropathy.

Promoting Mobility

Positioning

Change in position may also facilitate pain reduction. A new position can relieve pressure over bony prominences or areas of swelling. It can promote increased circulation, muscle relaxation, and general comfort. The client in pain may be reluctant to change position, fearing that pain will increase or damage will be done.

Immobility as the result of pain can cause multiple complications. It is important to teach the client how to change position safely and comfortably. Aids in changing position such as an overhead trapeze, bed rails, or arms on a chair are helpful. Use of pain medication or other adjuvant therapies prior to position change can further reduce discomfort.

Exercise

Exercise as a method of pain control is being investigated. Exercise, even gentle exercise, results in the release of endorphins, the body's own opioids. Endorphin release promotes natural pain reduction, as well as feelings of well-being. Exercise is also helpful in changing muscle tension, encouraging repositioning, and promoting increased function, such as when the client ambulates after abdominal surgery, resulting in an increase in intestinal peristalsis.

Energy-Based Approaches to Pain Management

Therapeutic touch and reiki are energy-based approaches to pain relief. Therapeutic touch uses the body's energy to promote relaxation and pain relief. Reiki promotes bodily, emotional, and spiritual harmony through precise hand placement on the client's body, resulting in increased pain relief. Both of these therapies promote a sense of warmth and well-being.

Acupuncture and **acupressure** are ancient Eastern techniques that involve changing energy flow through meridian or energy lines mapped throughout the body. Acupuncture involves the insertion of fine needles into identified acupuncture points, promoting balance and relief from pain. It requires the participation of a trained acupuncture practitioner. Insertion of the needles causes little or no discomfort. Acupressure involves exerting gentle continuous or intermittent pressure over identified pressure points, altering energy flow and promoting pain relief. It can be done by a healthcare professional or by the client after specific points have been identified and pressure techniques taught. Acupressure is also used in managing concurrent symptoms, such as when nausea is a problematic side effect of pain medication.

 Acupuncture should be used with caution in the immunosuppressed client.

Aromatherapy

Aromatherapy utilizes scents from essential oils to promote relaxation and relieve symptoms. Specific essential oils have specific uses, such as lavender for relaxation and tension reduction or ginger for nausea relief. The oil is placed in very small amounts on cotton or at strategic places in the environment. It can be used in healthcare facilities and taught to the client for independent use at home. This treatment modality is presently receiving much study.

Cultural Alternatives

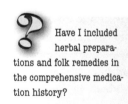 Have I included herbal preparations and folk remedies in the comprehensive medication history?

Cultural alternatives including the use of herbal remedies, cultural healers or practitioners, religious rituals such as prayer, and specific alternatives that have worked very successfully in the past should be incorporated into the plan of care. The healthcare provider can gain awareness of these methods through learning about the cultures or religions of clients served in a specific geographical area and through careful history-taking and assessment of the client and family. It is very important to be aware of the type of herbal remedies a client is using, as certain substances may enhance or inhibit medications being used, resulting in a change in the efficacy of these medications or presenting risks to the client.

Transcutaneous Electric Nerve Stimulation

Transcutaneous electric nerve stimulation (TENS) involves passing a mild electric current across the skin to superficial nerves near the location of the pain. Electrodes with positive and negative poles are placed on the skin and current flows intermittently across them, providing pain relief. Relief is temporary but recurs with repeated current stimulation. A small, battery-powered generator is used to provide electric current. This strategy for pain relief is initially set up by a healthcare provider but is usually controlled by the client and can be used in almost any setting. Despite the cost of equipment, it is cost efficient and safe, although some clients are reluctant to use electric current for therapy. It is especially useful in treating chronic pain conditions.

It is important when presenting physical and behavioral alternatives to clients to discuss them as complementary therapies. If the client perceives the strategies as an absolute replacement for medication, then pain management may fail.

BEHAVIORAL STRATEGIES FOR PAIN RELIEF

Behavioral strategies include intellectual, emotional, and psychosocial approaches to pain management. Their use can be extremely effective with a motivated client (and health caregiver) who is open to trying these somewhat unconventional methods.

Relaxation is a combination of physical and behavior methods. It can be achieved through controlled breathing exercises, visual or guided imagery, or progressive muscle relaxation. Relaxation reduces physical and emotional tension and promotes the release of endorphins. It also helps the client to feel more in control of the situation.

Meditation is a controlled, focused flow of thought that may also have a relaxing effect on the client and, through focus, help him or her to be more in control. Meditation is a learned skill; considerable client education and practice is necessary for success.

Biofeedback is a means of measuring muscular tension, electrical stimulation across the skin, and/or respiratory rate. Biofeedback provides concrete information to the client about his or her state of relaxation or arousal. Through successful use of biofeedback, the client can be more successful in reducing tension and anxiety.

Guided imagery can be useful not only in promoting relaxation, but in actual pain relief as well. Visualization of a special place such as the beach or mountainside is used in relaxation and as distraction from discomfort. Complex development of the image enhances therapeutic benefit.

It is essential to have the client participate in choice of image, to prevent biases or negative connotations from interfering with the process. For example, to ask a client who cannot swim to imagine floating on the ocean may result in increases in muscular tension and anxiety.

Proactive pain relief with guided imagery uses the imagination or an imaginary device to reduce pain. One strategy is to have the client visualize a meter and allow the meter to indicate present level of pain. It is a good idea not to become too elaborate in requesting the client to visualize this meter. Rather, allow the client to elaborate on what type of meter it is, having him or her describe it at length. Then, through imagery, the client turns down the level of pain on the meter, translating to less actual pain. Clients who practice this technique repeatedly can become quite successful. It is very useful for the client who must undergo repeated painful procedures.

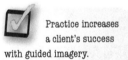 Practice increases a client's success with guided imagery.

Hypnosis and self-hypnosis have been used successfully in pain management. A trained hypnotherapist can place the client in a suggestible state and in this state help the client to manage pain or other adverse symptoms. It is very important for the client to understand that during hypnosis an individual cannot be forced to do something or divulge information. Not all clients are candidates for hypnosis. Those who resist it or are fearful of hypnosis and its consequences, even after receiving detailed information, should not be considered for this intervention. Clients can be trained to induce their own hypnotic state through self-hypnosis and to use this state of relaxation and focus to help reduce unpleasant symptoms.

Distraction from painful stimuli can be very successful in many client populations. Distraction can include simple interventions such as company, conversation, reading or television, or uncomplicated tasks. Distraction may also include participation in some ADLs. For example, many clients who are employed may bring work with them to treatment facilities. It is not unusual to see a client working on a laptop computer at the bedside. Engagement in activity provides distraction from pain.

 A wide variety of activities are appropriate for distraction therapy, and will vary from client to client.

Music therapy is a method consisting of active or passive use of music. There is evidence that music therapy can induce relaxation, moderate mood, and result in reduction of pain. Allowing the client to choose the type of music may increase success.

Music can be played in the environment or through earphones for only the client to hear. This has become a common practice during dental procedures. Some clients dislike the sense of isolation they get from wearing headphones, because they are then unable to hear what is going on around them.

Humor is an excellent alternative in managing pain. The act of laughing helps to generate endorphins and promote muscular relaxation. It can help reduce anxiety as well. Humor must be appropriate and not offensive. The client must be open and receptive to attempts at humor. Many facilities have instituted the use of humor carts, which contain humorous books, videos, collections of cartoons, and sometimes even samples of clients' own writings. Humor carts enable the clients to use this intervention on their own. When clients are part of a group, such as in an ambulatory treatment center or a long-term treatment facility, humor can become part of the group dynamic, used as a way to facilitate coping.

 Attempts to use humor must always be appropriate, respectful, and culturally sensitive.

Education

None of the behavioral therapies can be used successfully without client education. For this reason, adjuvant therapies have become

 When providing client education, it is important to remember that pain is definitely a barrier to learning!

the domain of the nurse as client educator. A plan for education, as well as assessment of learning styles and skills, for each individual client is necessary. Information in a variety of formats will enhance learning, as will multiple education sessions. Evaluation of material learned and reinforcement sessions will also enhance success.

Barriers to Pain Management

Through creative combinations specifically designed for each individual client, pharmacological, physical, and behavioral strategies can be effectively used for optimal pain relief. Client satisfaction with treatment and its effect on pain should always be the goal, and factors such as cost or healthcare provider attitudes should never be barriers to care.

Unfortunately, barriers such as cost and attitudes of healthcare providers can interfere with treatment of pain. Reimbursement for analgesics in health maintenance organizations (HMOs) is often limited to a few analgesics or NSAIDs. If these medications are effective and do not present a significant risk to a client, they may be appropriate. But medications on third-party formularies should not put a client at risk for a significant side effect or limit the potential effect the client could achieve with a drug that is not on the formulary because of cost. In short, cost should never be the determining factor for choice of treatment for pain.

Healthcare providers also need to consider optimal treatment plans without adding additional burdens. For example, analgesics such as acetaminophen and some NSAIDs are not available by prescription; therefore, they are not covered by most insurance plans. Despite the fact that they are not particularly expensive, lack of insurance coverage may make them an extravagance to some clients. It is vitally important to assess resource availability when suggesting use of an over-the-counter medication or any drug that is not covered by a client's insurance policy.

CASE STUDY RESOLVED

By the second postoperative day, Mrs. L. is ambulating with crutches. Her pain is well controlled with two Percocet (oxycodone 5 mg and acetaminophen 325 mg) tablets taken PRN every 6 hours. She is careful never to take them on an empty stomach. She mentions to the nurse that she has not had a bowel movement since before surgery. A bulk fiber laxative is administered, and the nurse instructs her to drink at least eight glasses of fluid each day. Her constipation resolves.

Mrs. L. is discharged to home on postoperative day 4. On a follow-up visit with her surgeon, she reports that her pain improved dramatically right after she returned home. "I think it was because I was so busy," she says. Three months after her surgery, she is completely pain-free in her right knee and has resumed all of the activities she enjoyed before her injury.

CHAPTER 3 · REVIEW QUESTIONS

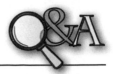

1. The most essential step in providing interventions for pain is:
    A. Medication administration
    B. Comprehensive assessment
    C. Client teaching
    D. Insurance coverage for palliative care

2. When selecting a medication for pain intervention, it is important to consider:
    A. That all medications work for all types of pain
    B. That narcotics or opioids are a better choice to relieve severe pain
    C. That choice of medication includes type, severity, and location of pain, as well as client-specific issues
    D. That medication is always the best choice to ensure relief

3. When utilizing opioids for pain management, it is important to also assess the client's:
    A. Heart rate
    B. Orthostatic blood pressure
    C. Bowel status
    D. Appetite

4. Use of multiple medications together in an attempt to provide pain relief is:
    A. Contraindicated because of multiple side effects
    B. Currently in experimental trials
    C. Useful only for severe acute pain
    D. Used when medications act in a synergistic fashion

5. The primary mechanism of opioids is:
    A. To promote sleep throughout the painful episode
    B. To bind with opioid receptors in the nervous system, blocking pain messages
    C. To promote muscular relaxation, reducing painful stimuli
    D. To induce amnesia, so the client will forget the painful episode

6. The most significant toxicity or side effect for which it is necessary to assess while managing pain with opioids is:
   A. Restlessness
   B. Respiratory depression
   C. Confusion
   D. Tachycardia

7. Neuropathic pain such as phantom pain after amputation is frequently responsive to which type of medication for relief?
   A. NSAIDs
   B. Opioids
   C. Nitrates
   D. Anticonvulsants

8. When considering a change from one type of narcotic medication to another for pain management, the nurse should consider:
   A. Equianalgesia
   B. Bioavailability
   C. Preferred route
   D. Equal dosing

9. The "gold standard" medication on equianalgesic charts to provide comparison is:
   A. Acetaminophen
   B. Morphine
   C. Codeine
   D. Meperidine

10. When planning for equianalgesia, which of the following must be considered:
    A. Medication to be administered
    B. Medication and route of administration
    C. Medication, route of administration, and times of administration
    D. Medication, route of administration, times of administration, and cost to the facility

11. A PCA pump would be an appropriate choice for which client:
    A. A 62-year-old woman with an elective joint replacement
    B. A 5-year-old having a tonsillectomy
    C. A 35-year-old having emergency vascular surgery
    D. A 62-year-old client with Alzheimer's disease

12. The client complaining of abdominal pain related to constipation would most benefit from:
    A. Opioid therapy
    B. Transcutaneous stimulation
    C. Dietary manipulation
    D. Ambulation

ANSWERS AND RATIONALES

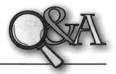

1. **B.** Intervention for pain relief cannot begin until a comprehensive assessment is completed.

2. **C.** Choice of medication for pain relief is dependent on multiple factors.

3. **C.** Opioids commonly slow intestinal peristalsis, contributing to constipation.

4. **D.** Multiple medications are used for both acute and chronic pain in an attempt to address multiple causes of the pain as well as providing enhanced effects through synergy.

5. **C.** Opioids bind with opioid receptor sites, blocking transmission of pain messages to the central nervous system.

6. **B.** Respiratory depression may occur with opioid use, resulting in a life-threatening oxygen deficit.

7. **D.** Anticonvulsants disrupt the afferent messages of pain.

8. **A.** Equianalgesia to prevent under- or overmedication.

9. **B.** Morphine is the "gold standard" for comparison.

10. **C.** Medication, route, and half-life of the drug all affect the choice when a different medication is chosen for pain relief.

11. **A.** This client would most benefit from PCA pain relief because of the opportunity for preoperative instruction on appropriate use.

12. **D.** Ambulation promotes the increase of peristalsis and the release of flatus, reducing discomfort.

REFERENCES

Acute Pain Management Clinical Practice Guideline Panel. (1992). *Acute pain management: operative or medical procedures and trauma. AHCPR Pub No. 92-0032.* Rockville, MD: Agency for Healthcare Policy and Research, U.S. Department of Health and Human Services, Public Health Service.

American Cancer Society. (2004). *Complementary and alternative cancer methods.* Atlanta, GA: Author.

American College of Rheumatology Committee on Clinical Guidelines. (2000). *ACR guidelines for osteoarthritis.* Atlanta, GA: Author.

Brant, J. M. (2001). Opioid equianalgesic conversion: the right dose. *Clin J Oncol Nurs, 5*(4), 163–165.

Karch, A. M. (2005). *2006 Lippincott's nursing drug guide.* Philadelphia: Lippincott Williams & Wilkins.

Management of Cancer Pain Guideline Panel. (1994). *Management of cancer pain clinical practice guideline. AHCPR Pub No. 94-0592.* Rockville, MD: Agency for Health Care Policy and Research, Public Health Service, U.S. Department of Health and Human Services.

McCaffery, M., & Pasero, C. (1999). *Pain: clinical manual* (2nd ed.). St. Louis, MO: Mosby; 1999.

Micozzi, M. S. (2006). Fundamentals of complementary and integrative medicine (3rd ed.). St. Louis, MO: Saunders Elsevier.

National Center for Complementary and Alternative Medicine. (2007). *NCCAM clearinghouse publications.* Silver Springs, MD: National Institutes of Health.

Snyder, M., & Lindquist, R. (2006). Complementary/alternative therapies in nursing. New York: Springer.

LEARNING RESOURCE

Sierzant, T. L., Portu, J. B., Belgrade, M. J., et al. (2001). *Pain management: an interactive CD-ROM for clinical staff development.* Frederick, MD: Aspen.

In the adult client, acute pain—pain which lasts for no more than 6 months—is often a problem. Acuity, in this case, refers to duration of the pain, not the severity. Acute pain in the adult has multiple causes and manifestations, and it is managed in many different settings. Causative factors can include trauma, cardiac and gastric disorders, childbirth, and chronic illness. Management can include pharmacological, physiological, and behavioral interventions. Greater success with pain management is common with the involvement of the adult client in the planning and implementation of pain.

4

Acute Pain in the Adult Client

TERMS
- [ ] acute pain
- [ ] adherence
- [ ] adjuvant medications
- [ ] behavioral intervention
- [ ] effleurage
- [ ] evaluation
- [ ] headache
- [ ] massage
- [ ] narcotic
- [ ] opioid
- [ ] pharmacological intervention
- [ ] physiological intervention
- [ ] plan of care
- [ ] self-management
- [ ] somatic pain
- [ ] superficial injury
- [ ] swelling
- [ ] transcutaneous electrical nerve stimulation (TENS)
- [ ] transcutaneous stimulation
- [ ] trauma
- [ ] visceral pain

CASE STUDY

Mrs. Y., a 42-year-old mother of three young children, is admitted at 8:00 PM to the emergency unit with an open fracture of the right arm as the result of a fall while skiing. She is awake and alert, and complaining of severe pain in her right arm. Surgery for open reduction and internal fixation is scheduled for the next morning, so the client is maintained NPO throughout the night. Her pain is initially treated with intramuscular meperidine (Demerol), with fair relief.

 ACUTE PAIN

Acute pain is a frequent problem in the adult population. Acuity, in this case, refers to duration of the pain, not the severity. This is an important factor to share with the adult client, as the word *acute* is synonymous with threatening or severe for many people.

Acute pain in the adult is commonly pain that is problematic for no more than 6 months. Pain continuing past this point is considered chronic, necessitating consideration of other assessment and treatment alternatives than those used to manage acute pain. In some cases, when the source of pain is identified, the pain may be diagnosed as chronic from the outset because it is the result of a chronic condition, such as rheumatoid arthritis. In other cases, the duration of the pain determines acuity.

 Acute pain: pain that occurs as the result of trauma, tissue injury, or illness. This pain lasts or is expected to last for no more than 6 months.

 Chronic pain: pain that lasts for longer than 6 months or is expected to last longer than 6 months because it is related to a chronic illness or condition.

 Severity of pain is not necessarily correlated to the type or severity of the traumatic event.

Causes of Acute Pain

Acute pain in the adult has multiple causes, manifestations, and is managed in many different settings. **Self-management** is common for the adult client with minor to moderate acute pain. Access to professional treatment usually occurs with increased severity of pain, accompanying issues such as open trauma, or when the pain interferes with everyday life.

Injury

One frequent causative factor in acute pain is **trauma**. A traumatic event can be work or leisure-related. It can be as minor as an abrasion as the result of a fall, or it can affect multiple systems, such as trauma from a major auto accident. Severity of pain is not necessarily correlated to the type or severity of the traumatic event. **Superficial injuries** that occur as the result of trauma are frequently associated with severe pain because of the large number of nociceptors present in superficial tissues. First- and second-degree burns are far more painful for the client than a more severe and destructive third-degree burn, because the third-degree burn or full-thickness injury destroys many of the nociceptors that would send pain messages to the central nervous system.

Visceral pain can also result from trauma, including trauma as the result of violence. **Somatic pain** is frequently reported, such as in a fracture or a sprain. Somatic pain is often associated with sports and physical activity.

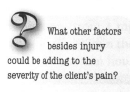 What other factors besides injury could be adding to the severity of the client's pain?

Illness

Medical reasons for acute pain in adults most commonly include cardiac and gastric disorders. In these instances, pain acts as a signal that there is impending or actual damage to the system. Pain related to a medical condition ranges from minor to severe, with no correlation to severity of disease or damage. It is very important for the healthcare provider to remember that pain is a subjective entity. One client may be incapacitated by pain related to gastrointestinal flu because the pain is perceived as severe, while a different client may continue to function in normal everyday activities through an acute inflammation of the appendix resulting in rupture. Although people often relate cancer to pain, pain is not commonly an early warning sign of cancer; rather, it is more commonly a later symptom of advanced disease.

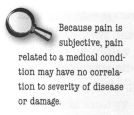 Because pain is subjective, pain related to a medical condition may have no correlation to severity of disease or damage.

Pregnancy and childbirth are responsible for acute pain, but this will not be addressed further in this chapter. Hormonal changes in females can be correlated with acute episodes of pain, including menstrual pain as well as midcycle pain associated with ovulation.

Multiple examples of acute pain exist in the adult population. **Headaches** are common in this client population. Headaches may be related to tension, hormonal shifts, and migraine. Sinus inflammation or seasonal allergies are implicated in episodes of acute headache. Headache pain is also described in certain individuals with a history of multiple or cluster headaches as acute episodes of a chronic condition. Dental pain is another acute complaint in this group. It may precede or be the result of dental procedures.

The healthcare provider has the opportunity to care for the adult client with acute pain in a wide variety of settings. Clients experiencing surgical pain are seen in inpatient and outpatient facilities, including ambulatory surgical clinics, private offices, and dental offices. Those with medical conditions are seen over the same wide variety of care settings. Long-term care facilities provide services for these clients as well. Most commonly, the adult client with acute pain is ambulatory and at least partly involved in self-care, taking active efforts toward pain relief. Healthcare access is sought when pain becomes a barrier to activities of daily living (ADLs). It is important to plan care and institute management with the input of each individual client, including him or her in providing for pain relief.

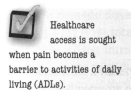
Healthcare access is sought when pain becomes a barrier to activities of daily living (ADLs).

 INTERVENTIONS FOR ACUTE PAIN IN ADULTS

Managing acute pain in the adult client can include **pharmacological**, **physiological**, and **behavioral interventions**. Except for mild pain, strategies for pain relief should include more than one treatment modality for optimal relief.

Pharmacology Interventions

Pharmacological choices may be over-the-counter, self-prescribed and/or self-administered medications, or narcotics with or without the addition of adjunct medications. Careful assessment of the pain for location, type, and severity is necessary prior to instituting relief measures. The clinical guidelines published by the U.S. Department of Health and Human Services offer a step-wise guide to the use of medication for acute pain.

Non-narcotic Medications

Mild to moderate pain may be relieved with the use of nonsteroidal anti-inflammatory drugs (NSAIDs) or other anti-inflammatory agents such as salicylates. These medications in common dosages can be administered on an as-needed (PRN) or around-the-clock basis. Using medication on an as-needed protocol sometimes results in increased severity of pain and reduction in relief, because the medication is not used frequently enough or is not used until the pain becomes quite severe. Complications or factors that may make pain worse, such as anxiety or muscular tension, may increase when there are long intervals between doses of medication used on a PRN basis, reducing the effectiveness of simple relief measures. Acute pain of more than a transitory nature may be relieved more effectively by using a NSAID on a regular dosage schedule, rather than waiting to re-experience pain before taking more medication.

Opioids

Acute pain that is not adequately relieved by these medications on a scheduled dosage protocol, or acute pain that is expected to be more severe, such as post surgical pain, can be treated with the addition of a **narcotic** or **opioid**. Choice of narcotic will include information about severity of pain, as well as client history of medication use and allergies. Codeine or oxycodone are common choices for less severe pain; morphine or meperidine (Demerol) may be used for pain that is more severe or not well relieved by codeine or a codeine derivative. Routes of administration for narcotics are also considered. Oral medication is appropriate for the client who is able to tolerate food or fluids. Intravenous medication is useful when the client must be maintained NPO (nothing by mouth), cannot tolerate oral food or fluids, or if extremely rapid relief is vital. Intravenous medications are cleared from the body much more rapidly than other routes, so administration must be more frequent to maintain adequate pain relief. Intramuscular, subcutaneous, or rectal routes are other alternatives. Transcutaneous administration is less commonly used for clients with acute pain. In clients who can tolerate oral medication, the addition of an NSAID to the narcotic regimen will increase efficacy. Oral preparations of codeine and oxycodone are manufactured in a form already in combination with acetaminophen (e.g., Tylenol #2, Tylenol #3, or Tylenol #4, and Percocet). One drawback of these combination tablets is that doses can only be titrated as high as the ceiling dose for acetaminophen. If further amounts of narcotic are necessary, plain codeine or oxycodone should be used. Overdoses of acetaminophen can result in liver damage.

Routes of administration may directly affect self-administration in the adult client. Ease of administration, as well as the client's ability to accept the route, are important to consider when planning care. Self-injection or relying on a family member to administer injections may be unacceptable. Many clients object to rectal administration as well, and family members often consider it undignified or embarrassing to administer rectal medications (e.g., suppositories). Timed-release oral medications, which restrict dosing to two or three times per day, decrease client burden and increase client adherence with multiple-dose schedules. Ascertaining that the client is comfortable with, understands, and is able to accomplish administration via a prescribed route is essential to client acceptance of a pain management plan.

Administration schedules for pain medication and adjuvant medications:
- **PRN:** medication is given at minimum hourly parameters upon the assessment by the caregiver that the client has pain or at the client's request (e.g., oxycodone and acetaminophen [Percocet], two tablets every 4 to 6 hours, PRN).
- **Around-the-clock:** medication given at determined or ordered hourly intervals throughout the day (e.g., oxycodone and acetaminophen [Percocet], two tablets every 6 hours).

Adjuvant Medication

In addition to narcotics and NSAIDs, other **adjuvant medications** may be added to relieve pain. These may include medications that reduce anxiety, promote relaxation or sleep, or reduce muscle tension. Assessment of the type and possible cause of the pain may indicate that some other form of medication is necessary for relief, such as medication for neuroleptic or anginal types of pain.

Adjuvant medications are drugs used in addition to the primary pharmacological intervention. They may use a different physiological pathway for relief, or may work in a synergistic fashion with the primary intervention.

Nonpharmacological Interventions

Physiological Interventions

Transcutaneous stimulation using temperature, pressure, or electrical impulses are useful in addition to, or sometimes in the place of, medication for relief of acute pain. Application of cold to the painful area results in slight numbing of the area. The sensation of cold is sent as a message to the central nervous system, short-circuiting the gate control mechanism for pain. Decrease in local body temperature results in slight vasoconstriction of the area, reducing local circulation as well as limiting the amount of extracellular fluid leaking into the area. Limiting extracellular fluid reduces or prevents swelling. **Swelling**, through increased local pressure, may thereby increase or even be a cause of pain. It is important to protect the skin when using application of cold to relieve pain. Ice should not be applied directly rather it should be wrapped in a towel or cloth. Cold should be applied intermittently. A good rule is 20 minutes on—20 minutes off. Continuous application of cold could result in tissue damage as the result of continued vasoconstriction. Clients who use cold or ice for comfort are often reluctant to remove it, because discomfort may recur with rewarming of the area. Therefore, client education is essential in using ice as a method of pain management.

Use of heat in pain relief is another common choice. Warmth often promotes muscular relaxation and a sense of comfort. Decreasing muscular tension may reduce pain sensations. Vasodilatation occurs locally in the area where heat is applied. This increases circulation, enhancing the removal of cellular debris, toxins, and extracellular fluid from the area of tissue injury. Although heat is not useful in preventing swelling, it is a great aid in reducing swelling that has already occurred. Reduction in swelling may enhance comfort. As with the application of cold, care should be taken to protect the skin where heat is applied. The older client or one with neuropathy is at risk for burns when heat injury is not noticed. Clients with mental status changes or who are sedated should also refrain from using heat for pain relief without supervision, as injury may result. Continuous application of heat is contraindicated for a variety of reasons. The same 20 minutes on—20 minutes off rule used when applying cold is a good idea. Increased circulation to the area may result in vascular congestion and weeping of extracellular fluid, actually exacerbating swelling. Temperature of any heating device, even a warm water compress, should be carefully checked to prevent burns.

Finally, heat should never be applied to an area where there is arterial vascular insufficiency. In this instance, metabolism and oxygen need are increased, putting the client in danger of injury from oxygen deficit (**Table 4-1**).

 When using heat or cold therapy to relieve pain, do not use continually or the client will be at risk for tissue injury. Instead, use the hot or cold pack for 20 minutes on, then remove for 20 minutes, then apply for 20 minutes, and so forth. Carefully assess the skin prior to reapplying.

Cutaneous stimulation in the forms of touch, pressure, or **massage** is another alternative for pain control. Simple touch or pressure applied continuously to one area or superficial massage short circuit the pain-sensation gate, sending alternate messages to the central nervous system. These can be useful even when the pain is not superficial. **Effleurage**, a gentle, rhythmic, superficial stimulation of the skin of the abdomen, is frequently used as one means of pain management during labor. Light massage or superficial stimulation may also reduce muscle tension and anxiety, and promote sleep. Deep massage reduces muscle tension but must be used judiciously when injury is suspected due to the danger of dislodging emboli that may travel throughout the circulatory system.

Massage may be a dangerous intervention, due to the risk of dislodging emboli, resulting in pulmonary emboli, myocardial infarction or stroke.

Transcutaneous electrical nerve stimulation (TENS) can be used to disrupt the pain message to the central nervous system. This requires

Table 4-1 Acute Pain in the Adult Client: Benefits of Heat and Cold Therapy

Cold	Hot
Prevent swelling	Reduce swelling
Reduce swelling	Increase circulation
Sensation of numbness	Promote muscle relaxation
	Decrease muscle spasms

particular equipment as well as input from a healthcare practitioner or rigorous client education before use.

Behavioral Interventions

Behavioral measures are another group of interventions used for acute pain management in the adult client. The client must be receptive and motivated to use behavioral interventions, and client teaching is necessary for success. Relaxation, visual imagery, hypnosis and self-hypnosis, diversional activity, and music therapy are some behavioral alternatives. Relaxation can be accomplished through breathing exercises—for example, those used in Lamaze childbirth—or through progressive muscular relaxation. These behavioral alternatives promote reduction of anxiety and muscular tension, as well as promoting rest and sleep. Successful use of behavioral techniques enhances the client's perception of being in control of the pain.

CASE STUDY REVISITED

During the night, Mrs. B. requests more medication than her q 4-6 hours PRN schedule allows. The nurse checks her arm, finding circulation, sensation, and motion intact below the fracture. When asked about the pain, Mrs. Y. complains that most of the pain is back pain. She has exacerbated an old injury in the fall. The pain is described as dull and cramping. The nurse assists to a more comfortable position in bed, applies a hot pack to the patient's back, and leaves her quietly watching television. When the nurse looks in 15 minutes later, Mrs. Y. is asleep.

CLIENT INVOLVEMENT IN PAIN MANAGEMENT

The adult client with mild, acute pain rarely accesses health care to manage the pain unless the pain interferes with ADLs or is perceived by the client to indicate a problem. It is more common for the healthcare provider to see a client with moderate to severe acute pain. Medication is the intervention of choice for moderate to severe pain. Transcutaneous or behavioral methods of pain management are rarely used in place of medication in the client with moderate to severe pain. Rather, such methods are useful as a way to increase the efficacy of pain medication or to reduce the amount of medication necessary for optimal comfort.

Involving the adult client in the planning and implementation of pain management increases the chance that the plan will be successful. This involvement includes client participation in the assessment process, a careful history, and client education in use of the alternatives chosen for pain relief.

Concepts of Adult Learning

The adult client has the ability to learn how to manage pain, but in this population, learning occurs differently than in children. Adults learn information more effectively if it is perceived as immediately useful and believable. The client who is not motivated to be a part of the pain-relief process or who does not believe that the identified options will be successful in relieving pain will learn less effectively. Barriers such as anxiety and discomfort also hinder learning, by inhibiting concentration

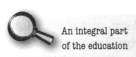 An integral part of the education process is to assess learning styles, and for barriers to communication or learning.

and recall. The client in pain, or one who is accessing the healthcare system, may suffer from varying degrees of anxiety. With this in mind, client education for pain management should be instituted prior to elective procedures that may result in intra-procedure or post-procedure pain. Measures to reduce anxiety will be effective in increasing retention of what is learned, as well as potentially contributing to pain relief. Some strategies for reducing anxiety include: providing information about procedures, the client's pain, and alternatives for pain relief; considering physical comfort in the environment where teaching occurs; and providing psychological comforts including privacy and support.

Adult clients learn through a variety of modalities. Spoken instructions or information are useful, but few clients are likely to retain all of what is told if the information is offered only once. Anxiety or pain reduces retention. Therefore, important information should be repeated, preferably several times. Information should be offered in small, distinct segments for better retention. Directions should be clear and concrete. Having the client verbally restate information or, even better, demonstrate the material being learned is an excellent way of assessing the success of the learning process.

Use of other means of communication increases learning. Providing written information as initial or secondary sources of information is helpful. Written material should be in a language that is easily understood by the client, without complicated technical jargon. Assessment of reading skill should be performed: never assume that a client has the ability to read. Pictures, demonstrations, and audio or videotapes are also excellent ways to share information. Including a significant other in teaching sessions may be helpful, as long as it is acceptable to the client and trust and confidentiality are maintained.

 Never assume your client is able to read! This assumption may prevent the client from obtaining information shared only in print format.

CASE STUDY REVISITED

Before her surgery, Mrs. Y. is visited by the nurse anesthetist who teaches her to use the patient-controlled analgesia (PCA) pump, which is meant to assist with pain control after surgery. In addition to explaining how and why the PCA works, she has also brought one to demonstrate how to activate the pump to provide a dose of medication on demand. She instructs Mrs. Y. on how to administer a demand dose and asks for a return demonstration. She leaves a printed pamphlet describing the PCA, which also has pictures indicating how it is to be used. She also spends some time teaching Mrs. Y. some controlled breathing and relaxation exercises.

 ## CREATING A PLAN OF CARE

After assessing the pain or potential for pain, creating a **plan of care** with client involvement includes documentation and sharing of intervention information. The North American Nursing Diagnosis Association (NANDA) classifications are one common method of nursing documentation, identifying, and defining client problems. A written plan of care is useful for easily sharing information with the client and with other healthcare professionals. The written plan of care also streamlines the evaluation process. Setting *realistic* goals for pain relief is very important. In many instances, complete absence of pain is neither realistic nor possible. Verifying client expectations and providing honest information about what he or she can expect will prevent failure.

 Are the client's goals for pain management congruent with the goals of the healthcare provider?

After assessment, the plan includes identifying measures for pain relief. These include pharmacological as well as nonpharmacological measures, considering availability of resources, and client receptiveness to offered alternatives. Medications that are appropriate for the type, severity, and location of the pain are identified with appropriate dose and route. Careful attention is paid to client allergy and medication-use history. Use of a medication that has failed to provide relief for this client in the past is rarely indicated. This would reduce the client's belief in the possibility of relief, as well as potentially reducing client acceptance and adherence with the plan.

Creative combinations of medication along with behavioral and physiological or transcutaneous alternatives increase the potential for success of pain relief. All aspects of the designed plan of care should be used for optimal success. The client should demonstrate understanding that components of the combination approach are not designed to be used individually, but rather that all components used together constitute the plan for success. Behavioral and physiological measures for comfort are not meant to replace the use of medication, although need for medication may be reduced by adding other types of interventions to the plan of care.

Client acceptance, satisfaction, and **adherence** to the plan are affected by the client's understanding of the plan, as well as the availability of resources and his or her belief that the plan of care will be successful. Even the most carefully considered plan of care is worthless if it is not utilized effectively by the client and other healthcare professionals. When identifying adjunctive methods for pain relief, consider the client's cultural and religious beliefs, which may indicate alternatives or restrict use of some already identified.

One creative way of increasing client participation and facilitating evaluation of the plan of care is through journaling. By encouraging the client to keep a journal of pain experienced and interventions utilized, information becomes available that will assist in modifying the plan. This can be a free-form written journal, a flow sheet, or a timed chart. Information to include in the journal would be occurrence (time), severity, and location of the pain; precipitating factors; and interventions used. Journaling improves client recall of pain and relief sensations. It is useful in tracking trends for relief and precipitating factors. It presents vital information for evaluation and plan revision. In the case of inpatient treatment with minimal client involvement or when the client is unable to journal, keeping a pain relief flow sheet or chart is a useful alternative.

Some clients report the act of keeping a journal is therapeutic in itself; it provides a greater sense of being in control.

Evaluation

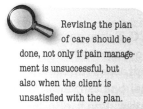

Continual assessment of the client's reports of pain as well as ability to accomplish ADLs should be used to evaluate the success of the plan of care. **Evaluation** includes revision of the plan when optimal relief is not achieved. An important part of client education is to offer and reinforce the idea that initial failure to relieve the pain does not indicate hopelessness. Reassure the client that multiple pharmacological and nonpharmacological alternatives exist for pain management and that continual evaluation and revision will establish an appropriate and useful plan of care. Encourage consistent client feedback in the evaluation process. In cases of difficult pain management, the healthcare provider should identify and utilize other resources, such as pain management specialists or clinics and review new literature. It is a realistic goal to strive for optimal pain management for all adult clients with or at risk for episodes of acute pain.

Revising the plan of care should be done, not only if pain management is unsuccessful, but also when the client is unsatisfied with the plan.

Consistent feedback from the client concerning pain relief and satisfaction with relief modalities promotes optimal pain relief.

CASE STUDY RESOLVED

For the first 24 hours after surgery, Mrs. Y. is quite uncomfortable. Although she is able to use the PCA morphine pump to control pain adequately, she suffers from severe nausea and vomiting. On the second postoperative day, the plan of care is to change her medication to an oral form. The nausea prevents this. The primary nurse knows that nausea and vomiting can be a side effect of anesthesia; however, it rarely lasts as long as 24 hours. She also knows that some clients develop nausea and vomiting when using morphine. Although this has not been indicated in Mrs. Y.'s medication history, she discusses it with the anesthetist, and the medication in the PCA pump is changed. The nausea resolves, Mrs. Y. is able to tolerate food and fluids, and on the third postoperative day her pain is well relieved by two Percocet tablets every 6 hours. She uses controlled breathing and relaxation exercises after physical therapy sessions.

CHAPTER 4 · REVIEW QUESTIONS

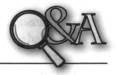

1. Signs and symptoms of acute pain include:
   A. Crying, grimacing, elevation in blood pressure and cardiac rate
   B. Flushing, tachycardia, fever
   C. Diaphoresis, pallor, bradycardia
   D. Stoicism, tachypnea, bradycardia

2. Causes of acute pain include:
   A. Trauma
   B. Hypoxia
   C. Bacterial infection
   D. All of the above

3. The process for managing acute pain in correct order includes:
   A. Evaluation, intervention, assessment
   B. Assessment, intervention, evaluation, reintervention if necessary
   C. Intervention, evaluation
   D. Assessment, intervention

4. Adjuvant medications are:
   A. Medications that do not require a prescription
   B. Medications given in conjunction with a pain medication to enhance relief
   C. Medications given in place of an ineffective pain medication
   D. Medications given to relieve side effects of a pain medication

5. Cold therapy may be used to relieve pain. When teaching a client to apply cold to an area, it is important to include the following information:
   A. Place ice directly to the painful area
   B. Use cold compresses or ice continually for 24 hours
   C. Do not apply cold to dependent limbs
   D. Apply cold to the area for 20 minutes on, then 20 minutes off; repeat

6. Use of heat to an area to relieve pain is effective because:
   A. Heat allows for increased uptake of opioids in the affected area
   B. Heat promotes muscular relaxation
   C. Heat promotes vasoconstriction, reducing swelling and local edema
   D. Heat promotes systemic vasodilatation

7. In a client education experience, anxiety or pain mediate learning in what way?
   A. They heighten awareness, allowing for increased retention
   B. They lower arousal thresholds, allowing for longer periods of learning
   C. They inhibit attention and reduce retention
   D. They decrease arousal, resulting in resistance to learning

8. A critical part of the plan of care to prevent or relieve pain includes:
   A. Careful assessment and history taking
   B. Formulation of a set of interventions
   C. Documentation of the plan to share with other healthcare professionals
   D. All of the above

9. Goals for a plan of care to relieve or prevent pain must be:
   A. Realistic and measurable
   B. Idealistic
   C. Attainable through the use of medication
   D. Involved and difficult to enact

10. When initial interventions are not successful to promote pain relief:
   A. It is important to reassure the client that other alternatives are available and to re-evaluate goals
   B. It is important to continue to use those interventions until they work
   C. A medical consult is in order
   D. Acknowledge that it may be impossible to achieve any level of pain relief

ANSWERS AND RATIONALES

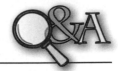

1. **A.** An increase in heart rate and elevated blood pressure are the usual manifestations of acute pain. Vital signs and other manifestations, however, may vary. At times, blood pressure may decrease with severe pain.

2. **D.** All of the above can be causes of acute pain.

3. **B.** Assessment is critical to planning intervention; intervention must be followed by evaluation, with further intervention utilized as indicated.

4. **B.** Adjuvant medications enhance the activity of a pain medication or target other symptoms such as anxiety and muscular tension, which may exacerbate pain.

5. **D.** Intermittent application of cold therapy to the painful area will prevent tissue damage, which could result from vasoconstriction.

6. **B.** Heat promotes muscular relaxation and comfort. It also promotes local vasodilatation, enhancing the removal of debris, toxins, and extracellular fluid.

7. **C.** They reduce the client's ability to attend to information, resulting in reduced ability to learn.

8. **D.** All of the above are critical to the formulation of a good plan of care.

9. **A.** Goals must be realistic for the client, the setting, the physical circumstances surrounding the pain, and for the healthcare provider.

10. **A.** Make sure goals are realistic and attainable, and reassure the client that if one set of interventions is not useful, other interventions targeting the cause or manifestations of the pain are possible.

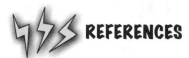 **REFERENCES**

Acute Pain Management Guideline Panel. (1992). *Acute pain management: operative or medical procedures and trauma. AHCPR Pub No. 92-0032.* Rockville, MD: Agency for Health Care Policy and Research, Public Health Service, U.S. Department of Health and Human Services.

American Society of Anesthesiologists Task Force on Acute Pain Management. (2004). Practice guidelines for acute pain management in the perioperative setting: an updated report by the American Society of Anesthesiologists Task Force on Acute Pain Management. *Anesthesiology, 100*(6), 1573–1581.

American Society of PeriAnesthesia Nurses. (2003). ASPAN pain and comfort clinical guideline. *J Perianesth Nurs, 18*(4), 232–236.

Institute for Clinical Systems Improvement (ICSI). (2006). *Assessment and management of acute pain.* Bloomington, MN: Author.

Karch, A. M. (2005). *2006 Lippincott's nursing drug guide.* Philadelphia: Lippincott Williams & Wilkins.

McCaffery, M., & Pasero, C. (1999). *Pain: clinical manual* (2nd ed.). St. Louis, MO: Mosby.

North American Nursing Diagnosis Association. (1999). *NANDA nursing diagnoses: definitions and classification, 1999–2000.* Philadelphia: Author.

Despite the multiple risks of surgery, the clients who are about to have surgery primarily fear pain: *"Will it hurt? How will I deal with it? How can it be treated or prevented?"* Pain is a common phenomenon in instances of surgical intervention and trauma. Although acute pain is a primary concern for surgical patients, two types of chronic pain are important to consider in the client who has had surgery: (1) pain as a result of the surgery, trauma, or illness, and (2) pain unrelated to the surgery that must be managed during the immediate postoperative period. The goals concerning surgical pain include management of pain prior to surgery, prevention of intraoperative pain or sensation, and prevention or relief of postoperative pain during recovery and rehabilitation. A wide variety of alternatives for pain management for the client with surgical pain exists, from medication of multiple types and dosage routes to traditional and nontraditional alternative therapies. Medications are very often prescribed for the surgical client. Comprehensive assessment and planning are necessary to manage a client's postoperative pain.

Opportunities for preoperative assessment and preparation for pain management are rare with increased movement of clients into and out of facilities pre- and postoperatively. Thus, the healthcare team faces two new challenges: timely and appropriate client education regarding pain management, and telephone triage to manage pain issues outside of the inpatient facility.

5

Pain in the Surgical Client

TERMS
- [ ] acute pain
- [ ] anesthesia
- [ ] anxiety
- [ ] chronic pain
- [ ] comorbidities
- [ ] complementary therapies
- [ ] conscious sedation
- [ ] deep vein thrombosis
- [ ] fluid accumulation
- [ ] general anesthesia
- [ ] hematoma
- [ ] ileus
- [ ] incisional pain
- [ ] inflammation
- [ ] informed consent
- [ ] neuropathic
- [ ] nonsteroidal anti-inflammatory (NSAID) therapy
- [ ] patient-controlled analgesia
- [ ] preoperative pain
- [ ] regional anesthesia
- [ ] somatic
- [ ] surgery
- [ ] swelling
- [ ] triage
- [ ] visceral

CASE STUDY

Mrs. R. is a 47-year-old woman who was admitted to an emergency department while on vacation in North Carolina, complaining of severe epigastric pain radiating to the right side, with nausea and vomiting. She reported consuming onion soup au gratin, quiche, and ice cream for dinner on the evening the pain started. Following blood work and testing, she was determined to be suffering from cholylithiasis. Her pain was controlled with meperidine, and she returned home to New York for an elective laparoscopic cholecystectomy.

On the morning of her admission, she is quite anxious about her surgery. After suffering severe pain with the onset of her illness, she fears that she will have severe, uncontrolled pain after the surgery. With this in mind, the plan of care includes admitting her to an inpatient unit for the night following her surgery, and using a patient-controlled analgesia (PCA) pump after surgery. The PCA routine is reviewed, and the admitting nurse reassures Mrs. R. that other alternatives are certainly available if PCA does not seem to be effective enough.

 ## PAIN AND THE CLIENT HAVING SURGERY

Pain is an almost universal phenomenon in instances of surgical intervention and trauma. **Surgery** is an invasive intervention with the intention of treating, controlling, curing, or stabilizing a medical problem. Surgery has many inherent risks, as attested to by the process of **informed consent** for both surgery and **anesthesia**. Despite these risks, clients who are about to have surgery primarily fear pain: Will it hurt? How will

> Invasive diagnostic procedures and surgery all carry the threat of pain before, during, and after the procedure. It is the responsibility of the healthcare team to assess, prevent, and relieve that pain.

I (the client) deal with it? How can it be treated or prevented? Surgical intervention is an alternative for most client populations, from the very young to the very old. The invasive intervention of surgery is even a choice for clients in special populations who require specific and different assessments and interventions for the resulting pain. It is a primary reason for admission to an acute care facility.

Surgery can be emergent in nature, unexpected, or planned. In these cases, pain management is purely postoperative. In other cases, the operative procedure is elective, allowing for a plan of care to prevent or manage pain, as well as client education in utilizing pain management techniques. Although prior preparation would seem to be the preferred alternative, it is a responsibility of the healthcare team to attempt to manage pain in either alternative. Surgical intervention is a choice of treatment for countless conditions. It is used to repair traumatic damage in the case of accident or injury, treat congenital anomalies, remove foreign bodies or disease, reduce inflammation as a pain-relief alternative, improve function, change appearance, facilitate childbirth, or as an exploratory or diagnostic procedure. An operative procedure may be curative, restorative, controlling, or palliative. Considering the reasons for surgery, as well as prior preparation and the personal meaning of the procedure to the client, are all-important in planning for pain management.

 Optimal management of surgical pain addresses preoperative pain, intraoperative pain, postoperative pain, and acute and chronic pain during rehabilitation.

 Lack of prior client preparation for postoperative pain management should not decrease the effectiveness of pain relief.

Preoperative Preparation

Historically, surgery was done in a hospital environment. The client was admitted to the facility, sometimes days before the procedure. The preoperative time was used for assessment, physical preparation, and client education. Recently, changes in technology and reimbursement issues have resulted in changes in where surgery is performed, as well as opportunities for preoperative assessment or client preparation. Now, surgical procedures may be performed in acute care hospitals or inpatient or outpatient units, in freestanding surgicenters, in physicians' or dentists' offices, in clinics, and in birthing centers. Minor surgical procedures previously done in the hospital, such as inserting central venous access lines, may now be done in a long-term care facility or even in the client's own home. When elective surgery is performed, even as an inpatient, clients are rarely admitted to the facility days prior to the procedure. Commonly, admission to the surgical facility takes place on the day of surgery through a day-surgery unit. Postoperatively, the client may recover on the day-surgery unit and go home that afternoon or evening or be admitted to an inpatient unit. In either case, opportunities for preoperative assessment and preparation for pain management are rare. With increased mobility of clients into and out of facilities pre- and postoperatively, the health-care team faces two new challenges: timely and appropriate client education regarding pain management, and telephone triage to manage pain issues outside of the inpatient facility. Client education will be discussed later in this chapter.

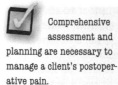 Comprehensive assessment and planning are necessary to manage a client's postoperative pain.

 ## TELEPHONE TRIAGE

Telephone **triage** is a method of assessment by phone used to evaluate the condition of the client, as well as provide appropriate interventions for presented client problems. It is a therapeutic exchange that requires the participation of a trained professional who can legally engage in assessment and treatment activities. It should not be left to an office secretary or answering service.

Triage is a formal procedure, with assessment parameters arranged to identify emergent or life-threatening symptoms and appropriate interventions, which may include activation of emergency services. Assessment criteria are also used to evaluate for less threatening problems. A triage manual with written protocols for assessment and interventions should exist for the practice. Complete documentation of each triage contact, including assessment, interventions suggested, client response, and resources used, is essential. A system for follow-up evaluation is also a good idea, and it enhances client satisfaction.

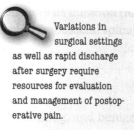 Variations in surgical settings as well as rapid discharge after surgery require resources for evaluation and management of postoperative pain.

Triage for the management of postoperative pain and potential complications should be available 24 hours a day, and it is imperative that the client and family are aware of how to seek out assistance from the triage service.

ACUTE PAIN RELATED TO SURGICAL PROCEDURES

Acute pain is pain that lasts for a relatively short duration, usually no more than 3 to 6 months. Clients rarely anticipate that operative pain will last that long. The goals concerning surgical pain include management of pain prior to surgery, prevention of intraoperative pain or sensation, and prevention or relief of postoperative pain during recovery and rehabilitation.

Preoperative pain is a result of disease or injury. Postoperative pain arises from a wide variety of sources and causes. It is important to evaluate and treat the specific types of pain during the pain experience.

Incisional Pain

Because surgery is invasive, most clients will complain of **incisional pain**, occurring secondary to impaired skin integrity from a scalpel or trocar entry into the body. Incisional pain can be quite severe, because it is cutaneous or peripheral pain. The skin and subcutaneous tissues have a rich supply of nociceptors, which readily transmit the pain message to the central nervous system. It is frequently described as cutting, searing, burning, or sharp pain. It can be more severe in certain areas of the body. For example, incisional pain is often quite severe in the axillary area following an axillary node dissection. Incisional pain can also occur in response to stretching or pulling of skin tissues during surgery and irritation from surgical prep solutions such as povidone iodine (Betadine®) or tape placed against the skin after surgery. Anxiety can also impact incisional pain, such as when a client manifests fear of disfigurement. The incision is usually covered with dressings immediately after surgery, and clients are often left to imagine what it looks like. With a fear of disfigurement, the incision and resultant scar can become a critical source of anxiety, reinforcing or exacerbating perception of incisional pain. Allowing clients to view the incision, as well as careful client teaching regarding the mode of closure (stitches,

Could anxiety be exacerbating the client's incisional pain, or are there signs and symptoms of complications of incisional healing?

Complications in incisional healing can be indicated by redness, swelling, hematoma or drainage at the incision, fever, changes in other vital signs, or increased pain.

staples, Steristrips), may help reduce anxiety in these situations, leading to improved pain control.

Surgical Pain

Somatic and **visceral** types of pain are commonly associated with surgical intervention. They are a result of surgical manipulation or removal of target organs for treatment purposes, as well as pressure from manipulation of surrounding tissues. These types of pain may also be related to **swelling**, **fluid accumulation**, or **hematoma** formation around the surgical area. Somatic pain arises in muscles, bone joints, ligaments, or fascia. It is structural pain and may occur at rest or with movement. Visceral pain is organ pain. It arises in the abdominal, pelvic, thoracic, or cranial cavities. Both are the result of stimulation of deeper nociceptors. Visceral pain can be diffuse and poorly localized; somatic pain is more specifically localized. Both may be constant or intermittent in nature. Client descriptions vary from sharp and severe to dull and achy. This type of pain is rarely described as burning or searing. It is the "expected" type of pain experienced after surgery or childbirth. Successful relief measures include a variety of pharmacological and nonpharmacological alternatives. **Anxiety** can also be a significant component in this type of pain, resulting in increased muscular tension with an accompanying increase in levels of pain.

Neuropathic pain is another type of pain frequently associated with surgery. It occurs because of surgical disruption or destruction of nerve fibers, either superficially on incision or deeper within the body. It can also be related to pressure or inflammation as irritants to the nerves in the surgical area. A client's description of neuropathic pain is usually characteristic—there is a hot, burning, or searing quality. Neuropathic pain is frequently resistant to common interventions for postsurgical pain and requires specific interventions.

Relief from neuropathic pain may result from medications traditionally used to prevent seizures.

Pain Unrelated to the Surgical Procedure

Many clients will complain about pain or aches that seem unrelated to the surgical procedure. Some common complaints include a sore throat, lower back pain, and limb or joint pain. Although it is important to assess each client who offers these complaints individually for signs of infection or injury, quite often these symptoms are related to the process of surgery. A sore throat may be related to intubation during anesthesia. A client undergoing a procedure including general anesthesia will often have an endotracheal tube placed to facilitate the delivery of anesthetic gases and oxygen, to maintain an open airway, and to protect from aspiration. The tube is usually placed after the client has entered an anesthetic sleep, and unless intubation and ventilation are required after the surgery, the tube is removed in the operating room or post-anesthesia care unit (PACU) before the client is aware of it. The irritation of the tube against the back of the pharynx may leave the client with a sore throat.

Back, shoulder, and limb pains are often the result of positioning during surgery. The operating table is a relatively hard, rigid surface with minimal padding. This is for both functional and safety reasons. After anesthesia has been administered, the client is positioned to allow the surgeon optimal access to the surgical area. Despite

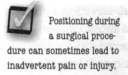

Positioning during a surgical procedure can sometimes lead to inadvertent pain or injury.

the fact that the client's body is padded and handled carefully and safely, these positions may cause muscle soreness postoperatively because of the long period of time the client has been maintained in what may be an awkward position on a hard surface. Clients who have orthopedic surgery, especially joint surgery, may complain of pain as a result of manipulation to position or seat the joint as part of the surgical procedure.

Back or shoulder pain may also be related to insufflation of the abdominal cavity with gas during abdominal or pelvic arthroscopic surgery. Although a major portion of the gas is removed by suction prior to final closure, some free gas remains in the abdominal cavity. Once the client sits or stands upright, the gas floats upward, exerting pressure on the diaphragm and creating characteristic shoulder and upper back pain. This is no cause for alarm, and repositioning may offer some relief. The client's body will safely absorb the gas in a short period of time, usually over the next 24 hours. Careful explanation about the reasons for these types of pain, as well as the commonality of their occurrence, may enhance other interventions for the pain.

Consequences of Immobility

After surgery, the client may complain of pain that does not appear to be directly related to the surgical procedure or to the processes described above. This pain is often related to the consequences of decreased mobility. Abdominal pain and cramping, especially of the lower abdomen, is a frequent complaint. It may occur in a client who has had abdominal or pelvic surgery or in one who has had surgery on a completely separate part of the body. The client who complains of this type of pain after abdominal or pelvic surgery is most likely suffering from decreased intestinal motility. Peristalsis tends to slow or completely stop (**ileus**) when the intestines have been handled or pushed out of the operative field. Assess for bowel sounds in all four quadrants, as well as for flatus and bowel activity since the surgery. In the absence of bowel sounds, the client should remain NPO. Decreased intestinal motility can also occur as the result of decreases in physical mobility, for example in the case of a client who has had orthopedic surgery followed by several days of complete bed rest. It can also be related to opioid use, which may result in retention of gas and constipation. This type of abdominal pain is not responsive to treatment with narcotics; in fact, narcotics may further slow intestinal motility and exacerbate the pain. An increase in the client's level of activity, with frequent ambulation, will enhance intestinal motility. Use of a cathartic suppository may also be considered.

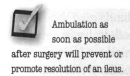
Ambulation as soon as possible after surgery will prevent or promote resolution of an ileus.

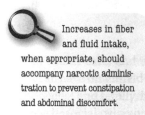
Increases in fiber and fluid intake, when appropriate, should accompany narcotic administration to prevent constipation and abdominal discomfort.

Leg or calf pain is another type of pain that occurs after surgery, especially when the client has been immobilized for a prolonged period. This pain may indicate a **deep vein thrombosis** (DVT), a potentially dangerous complication of immobility. The primary danger of DVT is embolization. The client who experiences leg or calf pain must be promptly assessed for accompanying signs of redness, swelling, and warmth to the area, as well as tenderness and fever. The client should immediately be placed on complete bed rest, and massage to the limb must be avoided. Application of moist heat may relieve the pain. With the diagnosis of DVT, anticoagulant therapy will be instituted.

Deep vein thrombosis is a potentially life-threatening condition!

Inflammation

Inflammation is a protective mechanism used by the body in a variety of circumstances to prevent injury to tissues and to remove foreign bodies or debris. It is primarily mediated by the immune system. Inflammation results in increased circulation to the affected area, with movement of fluid across vessel and cellular barriers. The consequences of an inflammatory reaction include redness (from increased circulation), swelling, heat, or increased metabolic activity and pain. Inflammation can be seen in the client as a normal response in the operative area or as a response to infection or allergy. It is a significant source of pain. The goal of maintaining comfort in the postoperative client has two components: to prevent inflammation and to reduce the inflammatory response, relieving the discomfort it causes. If the surgical area is peripheral, such as an arm or leg, maintaining the limb elevated above the level of the client's heart will prevent some swelling. Assessment for signs and symptoms of infection or hematoma formation allow for early treatment to prevent extensive inflammation. Hematoma formation is important because the old blood that accumulates in the area is an excellent source for infection, as well as a signal to the body for activity to commence to remove the debris. For this reason, surgical clients often have drains placed at the operative area. Heat and cold therapy are both used to help resolve inflammation and enhance comfort. Including anti-inflammatory medication in the pain relief regimen will also promote comfort.

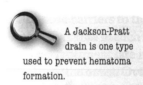

A Jackson-Pratt drain is one type used to prevent hematoma formation.

CASE STUDY REVISITED

Mrs. R. is admitted to the inpatient surgical unit from the PACU at 1:15 PM. The PACU nurse reports that Mrs. R. has ranked her pain as 3 out of 10 and that she is using the PCA appropriately. At change of shift, Mrs. R. tells the nurse that she has severe pain near her right shoulder blade "around a 6"; she is diaphoretic and her pulse and blood pressure are elevated. The PCA pump report documents that Mrs. R. has received all of the medication the program allows. After assisting Mrs. R. to a more comfortable position, the nurse gets an order from anesthesia for a bolus of medication and an increase in the programmed dose. Within

1 hour, Mrs. R. states she is pain-free and her vital signs have returned to baseline.

At 6:00 PM, Mrs. R. refuses her meal, stating that she is quite nauseated. Despite treatment with prochlorperazine (Compazine®) and ondansetron (Zofran®), Mrs. R. vomits twice and is very uncomfortable with nausea. The anesthesiologist elects to discontinue using the PCA pump and orders acetaminophen every four hours instead. Mrs. R.'s nausea resolves and her pain is well controlled using around-the-clock dosed acetaminophen.

 # CHRONIC PAIN IN THE POSTOPERATIVE PERIOD

Chronic pain has a longer duration than acute pain, lasting more than 6 months. It may be constant or intermittent. Chronic pain presents the challenge to the client of maintaining life in the face of pain. It is sometimes accompanied by decreases in mobility, capability for self-care, depression, and role changes. There are two types of chronic pain that are important to consider in the client who has had surgery: (1) pain as a result of the surgery, trauma, or illness, and (2) pain that is unrelated to the surgery but must be managed during the immediate postoperative period.

Chronic Surgical Pain

Chronic pain related to the problem that instigated surgery may be expected or unexpected. In some circumstances, it is not reasonable to believe that a client can become pain-free. In other instances, chronic pain occurs because rehabilitation and resumption of baseline levels of activity take longer than 3 to 6 months. Clients who have had aggressive orthopedic, cardiac, or gastrointestinal surgery often spend many months in the rehabilitation process. Chronic postoperative pain may also have a neuropathic element as the result of disruption or destruction of nervous tissue. Phantom pain, which occurs after amputation, is one good example. Chronic pain is often the reason for an elective surgery. Management of chronic postoperative pain is similar to that of other types of chronic pain. It includes establishing realistic goals with the client, frequent evaluation of the plan of care, and a commitment to managing this type of pain, which interferes with the client's return to baseline comfort.

Unrelated Chronic Pain

Chronic pain that is unrelated to the surgical procedure is a second challenge to the healthcare team. Many clients, especially the elderly, undergo elective or emergent surgeries with **comorbidities** that cause chronic pain. In addition to addressing surgical pain, assessment of baseline chronic pain and usual pain relief measures are necessary. In the case of osteoarthritis or other types of chronic pain, salicylates or NSAIDs may be the treatment of choice for the client. Medications in both of these classes can cause blood dyscrasias or clotting difficulties. Not only may clients be directed to discontinue use of these medications up to 2 weeks prior to elective surgery, but their use in the period directly after surgery may be limited as well. Acetaminophen is one alternative medication to replace these. In addition to medications, alternate interventions for relief should also be considered, including heat or cold therapy, exercise, and positioning as appropriate. Successful management of pre-existing chronic pain during the surgical period will contribute to a positive client outcome.

 ## SURGICAL PAIN MANAGEMENT

A wide variety of alternatives for pain management for the client with surgical pain exists, from medication of multiple types and dosage routes to traditional and nontraditional **complimentary therapies**.

Pain Management During Surgery

Pain management during the intraoperative period may be accomplished through the use of **general** or **regional anesthesia,** or with **conscious sedation.** Conscious sedation is a practice in which the client enters a state of twilight sleep but remains arousable and aware of his surroundings. An opioid for pain reduction and a medication that will cause amnesia during the conscious sedation period are usually included. The importance of conscious sedation during surgical or other invasive procedures is that pain is controlled and/or forgotten, but the client is able to cooperate during the procedure as well as maintain his or her own airway. Conscious sedation carries potentials for danger, including respiratory depression, oxygen desaturation, risk for aspiration, and injury. The client must be comprehensively monitored through the sedation period and until recovery is complete.

Postoperative Pain Management

Use of medication as intervention for postoperative pain is extremely common. According to the Agency for Healthcare Policy and Research (AHCPR) clinical guidelines for acute pain management, medication therapy should be a stepped approach. Mild to moderate surgical pain should be treated initially with **nonsteroidal anti-inflammatory (NSAID) therapy** (see Table 3-1 in Chapter 3). Acetaminophen may be the first drug of choice, despite its weak anti-inflammatory properties. Acet-aminophen is less likely to affect plate-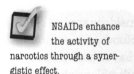 NSAIDs enhance the activity of narcotics through a synergistic effect.

let aggregation—an important consideration, as hemorrhage may be a concern after surgery. NSAIDs used alone frequently control pain well. Around-the-clock dosage every 4 to 6 hours is often more successful than administering them on an as-needed (PRN) basis. When the client waits until pain is significant to request or take pain medication, either NSAIDs or opioids, control of the pain can become difficult. Frequent assessment and evaluation of pain relief is necessary. Adjuvant methods of pain control can be added to the NSAID therapy. In the event that pain is not well controlled by NSAID therapy or pain is more severe, opioids can be introduced (see Table 3-2 in Chapter 3).

Opioids can be used in addition to NSAIDs but not necessarily as a replacement. Postoperative dose scheduling should be around-the-clock and not PRN for at least the first 36 hours after surgery. At this time, further assessment will dictate changes in scheduling or medication. Opioids can be administered through a variety of routes. In acute care facilities, when the client has established intravenous (IV) access, an IV route is chosen. The benefits of the IV route are rapid delivery of medication into the circulatory system and minimal invasiveness. Draw-backs include rapid metabolism and shorter optimum serum medication levels. The client experiences rapid, but short-term, relief. One excellent choice for many clients who are receiving IV medication for postopera-tive pain is the **patient-controlled analgesia** (PCA) pump.

A PCA pump usually connotes IV drug administration; however, in-tramuscular (IM), subcutaneous (SC), or epidural routes have been used with the PCA pump as well. The client who uses a PCA pump must be able to follow directions, willing to monitor and control his or her own pain, and motivated to take control. Ideally, client education about using the pump appropriately should occur in the preoperative period. Postop-eratively, pain, medication, anxiety, or anesthesia may interfere with the learning process; however, if preoperative education is not possible, it should not remove PCA as a valuable option.

PCA is administered using a programmable pump. The client is usual-ly given an initial loading dose (bolus) and can then request a determined dose of pain medication on demand. Demand usually involves pushing a small request button. The dose of medication, the minimum interval allowable between doses, and the maximum amount of medication al-lowed over a set period of time are deter-mined by the practitioner. Two alternatives are available: (1) the client receives a basal rate of medication, a continuous IV amount in addition to the client-demanded doses, or (2) only intermittent doses demanded by the client are administered. This is a safe al-ternative to intermittent injections of pain medication.

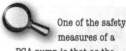

One of the safety measures of a PCA pump is that as the client becomes sedated from the medication, he or she does not push the demand button.

Drawbacks to PCA use include misunderstandings on the part of the client, physical or mental inability to use the pump, poor education or preparation for PCA as a pain-relief method, poor IV access, or reluc-tance on the part of the client to self-medicate for pain.

It is important to remind clients and their families that PCA pumps should be client-controlled!

Medications commonly used in a PCA pump may cause uncomfort-able side effects, including nausea and itching, or dangerous complica-tions, such as respiratory depression. Care should be taken to assess for and rapidly treat these problems. In the event of side effects that become a barrier to effective use of the PCA, an alternative medication or administration system should be considered.

Other routes of administration for postoperative pain medication include sublingual (SL) or transbuccal, rectal (PR), intramuscular, subcutaneous, or epidural. Transcutaneous administration of postoperative medications is usually not an option as it takes 24 to 48 hours to establish effective serum drug levels, and medication is difficult to titrate using this route.

For the client with mild to moderate pain, the oral route of administration is preferable, if possible. It is safe, easy, and economical. In the case of severe pain, oral use of opioids is one possibility; however, IV or epidural administration may provide greater efficacy. Changes in technology that have made pumps smaller, cheaper, and easy to use have made IV and epidural administration possible outside of the acute care facility. In many parts of the country, these routes of administration of medication for severe pain are even used in the client's own home with support from visiting nurses or ambulatory clinics.

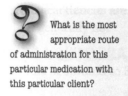
What is the most appropriate route of administration for this particular medication with this particular client?

NONPHARMACOLOGICAL CHOICES FOR POSTOPERATIVE PAIN MANAGEMENT

Pain management through nonpharmacological choices is important for the surgical client to use in addition to medications, as well as instead of medications. Choice of nonpharmacological methods should take into account the severity and reasons for the client's pain, as well as the client's motivation to utilize them. These methods are bound to fail if the client does not believe they will be effective or does not wish to use them. In assessing the client and planning for interventions, cognitive ability and awareness, cultural biases, and levels of mobility should be considered. A variety of cognitive or behavioral approaches are available, including relaxation, guided imagery, music therapy, distraction, and hypnosis or self-hypnosis. Ways to reduce anxiety and accompanying muscular tension will be useful. Physical methods of relief include light cutaneous stimulation and deep massage. Heat and cold therapies and exercise are also alternatives. All of these alternatives are described at length in other areas of this text. Careful choice of client education formats, including written, verbal, pictures, and video, can reinforce ways to use nonpharmacological methods.

In conclusion, comprehensive assessment and planning are necessary to manage a client's postoperative pain. Each client is seen as an individual with differing causes, responses to, and meanings for pain. It is an important goal for the healthcare team to proactively prevent severe pain in the postoperative period. Interventions may be more successful if the client has been included in goal setting and has received education about intervention methods. When possible, the most beneficial time to undertake this education is preoperatively, because pain, anxiety, and medications used postoperatively may be barriers to learning. These factors do no preclude or prevent learning but must be considered when client education occurs after surgery, as not all surgical procedures are elective and preoperative education may be impossible in many cases.

CASE STUDY RESOLVED

Postoperative orders include frequent ambulation on the first postoperative day. Mrs. R. seems reluctant to walk, even with the assistance of a nursing student. During her assessment of the client, the student finds out that Mrs. R. has suffered from chronic low back pain for years, which is quite painful. Her usual pain relief medication for this is ibuprofen, but she states she was told by her surgeon to discontinue use of ibuprofen for at least a week before the surgery. The nurse suggests use of warm soaks to the client's lower back prior to ambulation, which provide excellent relief. By afternoon, Mrs. R. is ambulating independently and ready to be discharged home.

CHAPTER 5 • REVIEW QUESTIONS

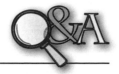

1. Assessment and consideration for pain management following surgery is best begun:
    A. In the post-anesthesia care unit
    B. Once the client returns to the surgical unit
    C. Only by a specially trained anesthesiologist
    D. At the same time as other preoperative assessments are instituted

2. Types of pain that are important to consider in the postoperative client when providing pain-relief interventions include:
    A. Acute pain
    B. Chronic pain
    C. Pain unrelated to the surgical intervention
    D. All of the above

3. Mrs. Smith is 36 hours postop following an abdominal hysterectomy. She describes abdominal pain as 7 on a scale of 10. It is cramping in nature and intermittent. Her bowel sounds are hypoactive and she denies passing flatus. The best intervention would be:
    A. Morphine sulfate 10 mg as ordered by MD
    B. Two Percocet tablets, PO as ordered by MD
    C. Ambulation at least twice per shift
    D. No intervention is necessary at this time

4. Incisional pain refers to:
    A. Mild pain experienced 6 to 8 months after surgery
    B. Sharp pain related to damaged nociceptors in the skin and subcutaneous tissues
    C. An allergic response to suture materials
    D. Insignificant, because it is only the result of anxiety

5. Clients complaining of back or limb pain after surgery are:
    A. Manipulating the nursing staff to get more narcotics
    B. Suffering from a phenomenon known as phantom pain
    C. Responding to the result of positioning during surgery
    D. Exhibiting signs of postoperative hemorrhage

6. Back or shoulder pain is frequently reported by clients who have undergone laparoscopic surgery of the abdomen or pelvis. This is the result of:
   A. Postoperative anxiety
   B. Placement of a nasogastric tube
   C. Incisional pain
   D. Trapped gas in the abdominal cavity

7. Mr. Allen is recovering from hip replacement surgery. Three days after surgery on his left hip, he complains of right calf pain. The right calf is red, warm, and tender to touch. An appropriate nursing intervention would be:
   A. To immediately place the client on bed rest with the right leg elevated
   B. To treat the right calf with gentle massage
   C. To apply ice to the right calf
   D. To increase ambulation

8. A 78-year-old woman is treated surgically for intestinal blockage. After surgery, ambulation is a priority to reduce complications related to immobility. Prior to her surgery, this client suffered from osteoarthritic pain of both hips and knees, which she treated with aspirin. An appropriate nursing intervention postoperatively would be:
   A. Use of warm, moist heat to the joints before and after ambulation
   B. Reinstituting aspirin therapy
   C. No intervention is necessary, as postoperative narcotics will manage that pain
   D. Vigorous massage to the lower extremities

9. To gain a postoperative client's cooperation in ambulating, coughing, and deep breathing, and turning, which is the most important intervention for the nurse to perform?
   A. Administer analgesics as ordered to ensure the client is relatively comfortable
   B. Be sure that the client understands the rationale for these activities
   C. Warn the client that life-threatening complications may arise if he or she is not cooperative
   D. Praise the client for completed activities

ANSWERS AND RATIONALES

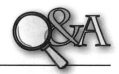

1. **D.** As other preoperative assessments are considered, it is essential to evaluate the client's pain history, as well as begin planning for pain management measures for after surgery.

2. **D.** All three types of pain identified should be considered in planning for the client's comfort.

3. **C.** Ambulation will promote bowel motility, relieving gas pains, which are most often described as dull, crampy, and intermittent. Use of a narcotic may actually exacerbate the pain by decreasing bowel motility.

4. **B.** Pain at the incision site is related to damaged nociceptors in the skin and subcutaneous tissues.

5. **C.** Usually, such aches and pains result from positioning or pressure during surgery.

6. **D.** Back or shoulder pain may be related to insufflation of the abdominal cavity with gas during abdominal or pelvic arthroscopic surgery. Once the client sits or stands upright, the gas floats upward, exerting pressure on the diaphragm and creating characteristic shoulder and upper back pain. Repositioning may offer some relief.

7. **A.** These symptoms would indicate the possibility of deep vein thrombosis in the right leg. To prevent potentially life-threatening embolization, it would be essential to immediately place the client on bed rest with the right leg elevated.

8. **A.** Use of aspirin directly after surgery is contraindicated, as it disrupts platelet aggregation, promoting the risk for bleeding. Use of warm, moist heat to the joints before and after ambulation is an excellent alternative for comfort.

9. **A.** Client comfort will promote compliance.

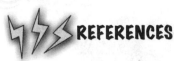

REFERENCES

Acute Pain Management Guideline Panel. (1992). *Acute pain management: operative or medical procedures and trauma. AHCPR Pub No. 92-0032.* Rockville, MD: Agency for Health Care Policy and Research, Public Health Service, U.S. Department of Health and Human Services.

American Academy of Ambulatory Care Nursing. (2000). *Ambulatory care nursing administration and practice standards.* Pitman, NJ: Anthony J. Jannetti, Inc.

American Academy of Ambulatory Care Nursing. (1997). *Telephone nursing practice administration and practice standards.* Pitman, NJ: Anthony J. Jannetti, Inc.

American Society of Anesthesiologists Task Force on Acute Pain Management. (2004). Practice guidelines for acute pain management in the perioperative setting: an updated report by the American Society of Anesthesiologists Task Force on Acute Pain Management. *Anesthesiology, 100*(6), 1573–1581.

American Society of PeriAnesthesia Nurses. (2003). ASPAN pain and comfort clinical guideline. *J Perianesth Nurs, 18*(4), 232–236.

Edwards, B. (1998). Seeing is believing—picture building: a key component of telephone triage. *J Clin Nurs, 7*(1), 51–57.

Fairchild, S. (1996). *Perioperative nursing: principles and practice* (2nd ed.). Boston: Little, Brown, & Co.

Girard, N. (2001). Clients having surgery: promoting positive outcomes. In: J.K. Black, J. H. Hawks, & A. M. Keene (Eds.), *Medical-surgical nursing: clinical management for positive outcomes* (6th ed., pp. 273–313). Philadelphia: W. B. Saunders.

Institute for Clinical Systems Improvement (ICSI). (2006). *Assessment and management of acute pain.* Bloomington, MN: Author.

Karch, A. M. (2005). *2006 Lippincott's nursing drug guide.* Philadelphia: Lippincott Williams & Wilkins.

McCaffery, M., & Pasero, C. (1999). *Pain: clinical manual* (2nd ed.). St. Louis, MO: Mosby.

Wheeler, S. Q., & Windt, J. (1993). *Telephone triage: theory, practice, and protocol development.* Albany, NY: Delmar.

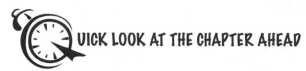

Individuals with cancer are at risk for a variety of physiological problems capable of causing pain. Comprehensive assessments for the etiology of the pain, appropriate treatment, and ongoing monitoring of pain are essential to achieve relief of pain and improve quality of life. Knowledge of the patterns of metastasis for cancer and the characteristics of pain are tools the physician and nurse use to identify the etiology of pain and subsequent treatment.

Changes in the nature and intensity of chronic cancer pain are critical assessment findings that require prompt medical treatment. Neuropathic pain often requires high doses of opioids along with adjunct medications to achieve relief and control of the pain. Although oral opioids and adjunct analgesics may effectively relieve neuropathic pain in some individuals, escalation of pain intensity may require rapid titration of IV opioids in a clinical setting that allows for close monitoring of side effects. Morphine continues to be the drug of choice for severe cancer pain, but high doses of morphine along with high doses of adjuvant analgesics are often required for pain relief and control.

6

Escalating Pain in the Adult with Cancer

TERMS
- ☐ epidural
- ☐ fibrosis
- ☐ intractable
- ☐ intrathecal
- ☐ morphine sulfate sustained release (MSSR)
- ☐ myoclonus
- ☐ neuroablative procedures
- ☐ neurostimulation
- ☐ plexopathy
- ☐ regional plexus
- ☐ regional infusion

103

CASE STUDY

J. T. is a 50-year-old patient with a 3-year history of lung cancer with metastasis to the bone. For several months, she has been experiencing pain that until recently has been well controlled with morphine sulfate sustained release (MSSR) (for example, MS Contin®) 90 mg PO every 12 hours and occasional morphine sulfate immediate release (MSIR) 20 mg q 2 hours PRN.

Two days ago, J. T. began to have more frequent pain in her right shoulder, which she rated a "7" on a scale of 0 to 10. Throughout the day she took six doses of MSIR 20 mg with good effect. The home health nurse contacted J. T.'s physician to request an increase in her MSSR to provide better pain control. The doctor ordered an increase in J. T.'s MSSR to 150 mg every 12 hours, and an increase in the morphine sulfate immediate release (MSIR) to 40 mg every 2 hours as needed. He also instructed the client to contact him if the pain continued or got worse.

One day after increasing her MSSR to 150 mg every 12 hours, J. T. rates her pain as "2" at rest. But the following day, J. T.'s pain rating increases to a "10" despite the increase in MSSR and increased use of MSIR. Today's assessment of pain indicates that the pain in J. T.'s shoulder is now associated with pain-

Is it essential that J. T. be hospitalized at this time? What should the home-care nurse do at this time?

ful sensations shooting down to her thumb and index finger. The nurse recognizes that J. T.'s pain is out of control, that it meets the definition for pain crisis as defined by National Comprehensive Cancer Network (NCCN) guidelines, that it is likely neuropathic, and that J. T. needs more aggressive treatment to control her pain. The nurse instructs J. T. to take a dose of MSIR 40 mg, and she contacts the physician, who agrees to have J. T. admitted directly to the oncology unit with a diagnosis of uncontrolled pain related to metastatic lung cancer.

THE PROBLEM OF CANCER PAIN

Surveys in the early 1990s indicated that pain was experienced by approximately one-third of individuals treated for cancer and more than two-thirds with advanced cancer. At that time is was estimated that in almost all cases (98% and 99%, respectively), clients should have had their pain adequately relieved. Instead, 40% to 50% of these clients failed to achieve adequate pain relief.

Since that time, there have been advances in the scientific understanding of pain, therapeutic options, and training of healthcare providers. Despite this, current estimates suggest that worldwide, as many as 50% of patients with cancer pain are inadequately treated. Table 6-1 addresses the steps required to improve cancer pain management.

 Cancer pain in the United States remains undertreated, despite a relative abundance of opioids, healthcare providers, and healthcare resources. In poorer nations, cancer pain is undertreated because of the lack of available morphine.

The purpose of this chapter is to educate current and future healthcare providers about clinical problems in the management of pain that they may not encounter in traditional curricula. Hopefully it will enlighten providers in such a way that improvements in the management of cancer pain occur and more relief is achieved.

TYPES OF CANCER PAIN

Etiologies of Cancer Pain

Pain related to cancer can be classified according to its etiology, its origin and character, and its duration. Cancer pain can be secondary to:

1. Tumor involvement;
2. Cancer-related procedures and treatment effects; or
3. Causes unrelated to cancer or its treatment.

Pain associated with a tumor is responsible for the majority of pain related to cancer. An example of this type of pain would be abdominal pain related to a colorectal tumor obstructing the large colon. Nerve damage secondary to chemotherapy resulting in peripheral neuropathy is an example of pain related to cancer therapy. Pain related to appendicitis is an example of pain unrelated to cancer or the treatment.

Table 6-1   What is Needed to Improve Management of Cancer Pain

- Improved physician/nursing skill in comprehensive pain assessment
- Collaboration of clinicians with pain and palliative care consultants
- Use of existing computer resources
- Individual accountability
- Systemic Monitoring

Note: From: The Grossman/Dunbar/Nesbit Article Reviewed. J. Abrahm. 2006. *Oncology.* pp. 1340–1342.

Origins of Cancer Pain

Cancer pain can also be classified according to its origin and character. Nociceptive pain refers to pain that is directly related to tumor infiltration of either somatic (for example, joint, muscle, bone) or visceral (for example, gastrointestinal tract) structures. Somatic pain is characterized as well-localized, deep, dull, or achy. The underlying cause is usually an inflammatory process. Bone metastasis, incisional pain, and wound pain are examples of somatic pain. Visceral pain originating from gastrointestinal tract structure is characterized as poorly localized, vague pressure that is often constricting or cramping. Visceral pain is often present in clients with advanced colon, pancreatic, ovarian, or uterine cancers secondary to stretching of the mesentery and abdominal organs.

Neuropathic pain applies to a variety of pain syndromes characterized by aberrant or somatosensory processes that originate in the peripheral or central nervous system. It is described as sharp, tingling, burning, shooting, shock-like, or electric. Sources of neuropathic pain involve tumor invasion of nerves, post-herpetic neuralgia, chemical damage to nerves from chemotherapy, surgical interruption of nerves, or spinal nerve root compression.

Duration of Cancer Pain

Cancer pain is also classified in terms of duration, with acute pain generally being defined as lasting less than 6 months and chronic pain lasting longer than 6 months. Pain related to an unresectable or recurrent tumor is generally chronic in duration.

Pain that occurs intermittently in clients with chronic cancer pain may be described as episodic. Episodic pain can be categorized in three distinct ways: incident pain, end-of-dose pain, and breakthrough pain.

Incident pain is related to a particular activity or experience, such as getting out of bed or reacting to emotional stimuli such as fear. End-of-dose pain occurs when the effect of a long-acting analgesic is not sustained over an expected duration. Breakthrough pain is a transitory episode of pain that is rapid in onset and usually of short duration (< 30 minutes). Breakthrough pain may occur despite adequate titration of long-acting opioids or continuous intravenous (IV) opioid drips.

SEVERITY OF CANCER PAIN

The intensity of chronic cancer pain varies from mild (1–3) to moderate (4–6) to severe or excruciating (7–10). Most clients describe their cancer pain as mild to moderate (1–6). If an increase in the intensity of chronic cancer pain occurs, prompt medical attention is warranted to fully assess the pain and determine its origin. Increased pain often represents progression of cancer, particularly in advanced disease. However, new pain in a person with cancer may also be a sign of infection, fracture, or a neurological problem. It is essential that client reports of a "new" pain be thoroughly explored to ensure that a reversible complication (such as spinal cord compression) is not overlooked. Reports of pain, especially of increased severity or at a new location, must not automatically be attributed to a pre-existent cause or to opioid tolerance. Opioid tolerance is seldom the cause of increased cancer pain.

Knowledge of relationships that certain cancers have with pain patterns and patterns of metastasis helps determine the etiology of new pain. Multiple myeloma and cancers of the breast, prostate, and lung account for the majority of cancers with bone metastasis that frequently is characterized by pain. Pain in bones is caused by direct tumor involvement of bone with activation of nociceptors or from compression of adjacent nerves, vascular structures, and soft tissue. With multiple sites involved, clients with bone metastasis commonly have multiple areas of pain. Complications of bone metastasis, such as pathological fractures or spinal cord compression, can lead to additional sources for pain and morbidity. Spinal cord or epidural compression commonly occurs with cancers of the breast, prostate, lung, and kidney, as well as with multiple myeloma and melanoma.

Plexopathies caused by an infiltration of nerves by the tumor or compression of nerves by **fibrosis** are another source of cancer-related pain. Cervical plexopathy is commonly related to primary head and neck cancers with local metastasis. Brachial plexopathy is commonly related to lymphoma or cancer of the breast and lung. Lumbosacral plexopathy can occur by direct spread from sarcomas, lymphomas, and colorectal, endometrial, and renal cancers. Peripheral neuropathy related to cancer pain can occur when peripheral nerves are infiltrated by tumor or constricted by fibrosis. Multiple myeloma causes a peripheral neuropathy in about 15% of clients. Peripheral nerves can also be damaged by neurotoxic chemotherapy (such as vincristine, cisplatin, and paclitaxel [Taxol®]), and after cutaneous incisions and retraction of tissues during surgery.

Neuralgia resulting from infection or reactivation of varicella-zoster virus is another cause of pain related to cancer. This neuralgia can cause both acute and chronic pain, which commonly affect thoracic and cranial dermatomes.

 TREATMENT OF CANCER PAIN

Treatment of cancer pain in adults should be guided by the clinical practice guideline developed by the National Comprehensive Cancer Network (NCCN) Adult Cancer Pain panel. This guideline is unique in that it acknowledges the range of complex decisions faced in caring for patients with pain. It is particularly helpful when dealing with patients with uncontrolled or escalating pain.

The NCCN guideline uses an algorithm that distinguishes three levels of pain intensity, based on a 0–10 numerical rating scale, with 10 being the worst pain: severe pain being 7–10; moderate pain 4–6; and mild pain 1–3). Mild pain (1–3) can be treated with a nonsteroidal anti-inflammatory drug (NSAID) or acetaminophen if the patient is not on analgesics, or a short-acting opioid. Moderate pain (4–6) is treated with a short-acting opioid, which may be titrated to effect. Severe pain (7–10), which is considered a pain emergency, is treated with a short-acting opioid, which is rapidly titrated for relief of pain. Morphine sulfate immediate release (MSIR) given orally or intravenously is commonly used as a short-acting opioid for pain.

Morphine injections via the subcutaneous or intramuscular route are avoided because they cause pain and because variations in absorption make it difficult to titrate medication to achieve a steady state of analgesia. Incident pain, such as pain related to movement, may be treated prophylactically prior to an event (for example, getting out of bed). End-of-dose pain generally requires an increase in around-the-clock or long-acting opioids.

Chronic cancer pain is ideally treated with around-the-clock medication to maintain a consistent blood level of analgesic, with the goal of preventing episodes of pain. To achieve a consistent level of analgesic, clients with chronic cancer pain who are able to swallow oral medications are treated with regular dosing of an immediate-release opioid for at least 48 hours. Once the patient has demonstrated the ability to safely tolerate around-the-clock opioids, the prescriber considers initiating a long-acting opioid such as **morphine sulfate sustained release (MSSR or MS Contin®)** or sustained-release oxycodone (Oxycontin SR®). If a client is unable to safely swallow a long-acting oral preparation, he or she may be a candidate for transdermal fentanyl. However, when transdermal fentanyl is started, therapeutic effect of the drug is not achieved for 12 to 16 hours. For this reason, a switch to transdermal fentanyl is usually appropriate only when pain is well controlled.

CASE STUDY REVISITED

The escalation of J. T.'s pain is thought to be related to metastasis of her lung cancer to the brachial plexus. The diagnosis of this new pain source is facilitated by J. T.'s description that the pain feels like a shooting, electric sensation in her thumb and index finger that begins in the right shoulder. Knowledge that this pain likely represents the neuropathic pain characteristic of brachial plexopathy and understanding of the relationship of brachial plexopathy with lung cancer may prompt the physician to validate the diagnosis by computed tomography. However, effective treatment of the pain with verbalized relief by the patient is the priority.

An increase in pain may represent progression of the cancer, particularly in advanced disease. However, new pain in a person with cancer may also be a sign of infection, fracture, or a neurological problem, which may be reversible.

TREATMENT OF NEUROPATHIC PAIN RELATED TO CANCER

Neuropathic pain is considered one of the most difficult types of pain to control. Although it is less responsive to opioids than nociceptive pain, opioids are the first line of treatment for cancer related neuropathic pain, with morphine sulfate (or equivalent) the drug of choice. Because neuropathic pain is less responsive to opioids, higher doses are generally required for its relief and control.

Opioids have a wide range of effects, and their effectiveness is dependent on the individual's particular response to the drug. Thus, one person's pain might respond well to a low dose of opioid, which may provide little, if any, effect for another's pain. When using opioids without a ceiling dose, the amount of the drug that the person requires for relief and control of pain is not as important as is the individual's ability to tolerate side effects. Increases in opioids (without a ceiling dose) for uncontrolled cancer pain are acceptable as long as there is a balance between the medication's beneficial effect and its adverse effects.

Although respiratory depression is a potential risk when opioid doses are increased, it has not been found to be a common problem for individuals who have been receiving opioids for a long period of time or for clients with excruciating pain. Sedation as a side effect tends to be a more common reason for limiting opioids in clients with chronic cancer. Nausea can be another dose-limiting factor for use of opioids. Intermittent or around-the-clock doses of antiemetics can often be given to prevent or treat nausea or vomiting. Nausea related to narcotics also can be temporary, subsiding within a few days of opioid increases. However, nausea and vomiting, as well as other side effects, may be unmanageable when opioid doses are increased. If a client has unmanageable side effects on a high dose of one opioid, the recommendation is to change to a different opioid.

Neuropathic pain that does not respond to opioids is often treated with a trial of an antidepressant such as nortiptyline (Pamelor®), doxepin (Sinequan®), desipramine (Norpramin®), venlafaxine (Effexor®), or duloxetine (Cymbalta®). A trial of anticonvulsants such as gabapentin, carbamazepine, or pregabalin could also be undertaken. Both antidepressants and anticonvulsants are started at a low dose, and increased every three to five days, if tolerated. Topical agents such as capsaicin and local anesthetics including a lidocaine patch may also be considered (**Table 6-2**).

Table 6-2 Adjuvant Analgesics for Neuropathic Cancer Pain

Class	Generic Name	Trade Name
Antidepressants	Nortriptyline	Pamelor
	Doxepin	Sinequan
	Desipramine	Norpramin
	Venlafaxine	Effexor
	Duloxetine	Cymbalta
Anticonvulsants	Gabapentin	Neurontin
	Carbamazepine	Tegretol
	Pregabalin	Lyrica
Local anesthetics	Lidocaine	Xylocaine
Corticosteroids	Dexamethasone	Decadron
	Prednisone	Deltasone
Miscellaneous	Capsaicin cream	Capzasin P

Healthcare providers who are not knowledgeable about pain management are often reluctant to order adjuvant medications. This reluctance increases the risk that cancer pain will be poorly controlled.

If nerve compression or inflammation is contributing to the pain, a trial of corticosteroids can also be implemented. These medications can relieve neuropathic pain by reducing edema that occurs with compression of nervous system structures. Steroids such as dexamethasone (Decadron®) or prednisone are recommended with opioids for the management of pain caused by brachial or lumbosacral plexopathy. Steroids are typically given in high doses during acute episodes of severe pain, then quickly tapered to avoid long-term side effects.

Clients who are unable to tolerate adequate amounts of analgesia should be referred to a specialist who is skilled in more invasive approaches to the management of pain. **Regional infusion** of analgesics (**epidural**, **intrathecal**, and **regional plexus**) allows higher amounts of analgesic to be delivered to the source of the pain, decreasing or eliminating the systemic effects that occur with oral or IV delivery. **Neuroablative**

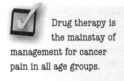

Drug therapy is the mainstay of management for cancer pain in all age groups.

procedures and **neurostimulation** procedures may also be appropriate.

CASE STUDY RESOLVED

After receiving the order for J. T.'s admission to the hospital, the home-care nurse coordinates her transfer. Because her pain increases with movement, the decision is made to arrange for an ambulance to transfer her via a stretcher, which will minimize her movement, and consequently her pain. The nurse assesses how long it has been since J. T. last took MSIR. J. T. states she has not taken any morphine for 2 hours, and she denies having taken more than one dose (40 mg) every 2 hours through the night. Recognizing that J. T. is not oversedated, that she does not likely have respiratory depression, that she has severe pain, and that it would take at least 30 minutes before she would be given analgesia in the hospital, the nurse instructs J. T. to take another dose (40 mg) prior to transfer to the hospital, and to take her MSIR with her to the hospital. The nurse then calls the oncology unit to give a report on J. T., emphasizing the need for prompt treatment and control of the **intractable** pain.

On arrival to the emergency department, an intravenous saline lock is inserted to administer analgesia with rapid onset of action. Analgesics given IV push will have a short half-life and will be quickly metabolized to decrease the risk of toxicity. Analgesics for J. T. are ordered according to the cancer pain emergency protocol that guides the physicians and nurses in aggressive yet safe treatment for severe pain. The protocol calls for the assessment of pain intensity (using a 0 to 10 rating scale), vital signs and level of consciousness. The patient is also assessed for possible nausea, itching, and **myoclonus** (twitching).

The protocol used for J. T. is based on the NCCN Adult Cancer Pain Guidelines, which recommend the following initial intravenous loading dose of opioids for patients in pain crisis:

- For patients currently taking opioids, give a dose increase of 10% of daily IV morphine equivalent to what the patient is currently taking.
- For patients not taking opioids, give 1–5 mg of IV morphine sulfate equivalent.
- The patient is reassessed for efficacy and side effects every 15 minutes to calculate subsequent doses of opioids. If the pain score remains unchanged or increased, the opioid dose is doubled. If inadequate response is seen after 2-3 cycles, alternate strategies can be considered.
  - If the pain score decreases to 4–6, the same dose of opioid is repeated and reassessment is performed at 15 minutes.
  - If the pain decreases to 0–3, the current effective dose of opioid is administered as needed.

Soon after arrival to the Oncology Unit, J. T. rates her pain "10" and is given morphine sulfate 10 mg IV. Fifteen minutes later she rates her pain a "6," is awake, with respiratory rate of 14, and no twitching. Morphine sulfate 10 mg IV is repeated; fifteen minutes later, J. T. states her pain is only barely present, and rates it as "1." She states she is very comfortable, and thinks she would like to sleep. The physician orders that she be started on a continuous IV morphine drip at 6 mg per hour, with a bolus dose of 3 mg IV PRN every 20 minutes. J. T. is monitored closely for adequacy of pain relief and development of adverse side effects.

A physician with expert knowledge in the treatment of neuropathic pain will evaluate J. T.'s plan of care prior to discharge. If her pain remains well controlled, she may be able to be started on oral analgesics and weaned off of the intravenous drip.

The decision to hospitalize the patient for out-of-control pain is up to the physician and the patient, and is determined by patient preference, intensity of the pain, time required to implement a plan of care, functional status prognosis of the patient, and need for monitoring. If the patient prefers to stay at home, the home-care nurse will need to consider the agency's ability to promptly deliver, initiate, and maintain morphine or another analgesic through a patient-controlled analgesia (PCA) pump for intravenous administration. If the patient who wants to stay home has a prognosis of 6 months or less, hospice services should be considered.

CHAPTER 6 • REVIEW QUESTIONS

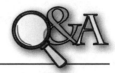

1. Of the following, which would most likely cause neuropathic pain?
    A. Bone metastasis
    B. Bowel obstruction
    C. Brachial plexopathy
    D. Brain tumor

2. Breakthrough pain in clients with chronic cancer should be treated with:
    A. Long-acting analgesics
    B. Short-acting analgesics
    C. Analgesics with a long half-life
    D. Adjuvant medications

3. Which of the following side effects occurs most often when opioids are increased for chronic cancer pain?
    A. Respiratory depression
    B. Sedation
    C. Vomiting
    D. Opioid toxicity

4. Which of the following adjunct medications is an antidepressant that is commonly used for neuropathic pain?
    A. Acetaminophen
    B. Nortriptyline
    C. Dexamethasone
    D. Phenytoin

ANSWERS AND RATIONALES

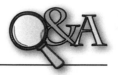

1. **C.** The brachial plexus is a network of nerves in the neck passing under the clavicle and into the axilla. Plexopathies cause neuropathic pain.

2. **B.** Breakthrough pain requires an opioid that works quickly.

3. **B.** Sedation is a common side effect of opioids. Although respiratory depression is a potential risk when opioids are increased, it has not been found to be a common problem for people who have been receiving opioids for chronic pain. Vomiting and/or opioid toxicity can occur but are not as common an occurrence as sedation.

4. **B.** Nortriptyline is an antidepressant used as an adjuvant for neuropathic pain. Acetaminophen is an analgesic. Dexamethasone is a corticosteroid, often used in pain for its antiinflamatory effect. Phenytoin is an anticonvulsant.

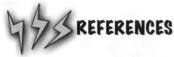

REFERENCES

Abrahm, J. (2006). The Grossman/Dunbar/Nesbit Article Reviewed. *Oncology, 20*(11), 1340–1342.

American Pain Society. (2003). Principles of analgesic use in the treatment of acute pain and cancer pain (5th ed.). Glenview, IL: Author.

Azevedo São Leão Ferreira, K., Kimura, M., & Jacobsen Teixeira, M. (2006). The WHO analgesic ladder for cancer pain control, twenty years of use. How much pain relief does one get from using it? *Support Care Cancer, 14*(11), 1086–1093.

Cabaleiro, J. (2002). Assessing and treating neuropathic pain. *Home Healthcare Nurse, 20*(11), 718–723.

Cherny, N., & Portenoy, R. (1994).The management of cancer pain. *CA Cancer J Clinicians, 44*, 262–303.

Coluzzi, P. (1998). Cancer pain management: newer perspectives on opioids and episodic pain. *Am J Hospice Palliative Care, 15*, 13–22.

Coyle, N., & Layman-Goldstein, M. (2006). Pain assessment and pharmacological interventions. In M. L. Matzo & D. W. Sherman (Eds.), *Palliative care nursing: quality care to the end of life.* (2nd ed., pp. 345–406). New York: Springer.

Grossman, S. A., Dunbar, E. M., & Nesbitt, S. A. (2006). Cancer pain management in the 21st century. *Oncology, 20*, 1333–1340.

Hagen, N. A., Elwood, T., & Ernst, S. (1997). Cancer pain emergencies: a protocol for management. *J Pain Symptom Mgt, 14*, 45–50.

Koshy, R. C., Rhodes, D., Devi, S., et al. (1998). Cancer pain management in developing countries: A mosaic of complex issues resulting in inadequate analgesia. *Support Care Cancer, 6*(5), 430–437.

Management of Cancer Pain Guidelines Panel. (1994). *Managing Cancer Pain Clinical Practice Guideline.* AHCPR Pub No. 94-0595. Rockville, MD: Agency for Health Care Policy and Research, Public Health Service, U.S. Department of Health and Human Services.

Mickle, J. (2002). Cancer pain management. In B. St. Marie (Ed.), *Core curriculum for pain management nursing* (pp. 349–366). Philadelphia: Saunders.

National Comprehensive Cancer Network, *NCCN adult cancer pain clinical practice guidelines in oncology, v.1.2007.* Retrieved July 31, 2007 from www.nccn.org.

Serlin, R. C., Mendoza, T. R., Nakamura, Y., et al. (1995). When is cancer pain mild, moderate or severe? Grading pain severity by its interference with function. *Pain, 61*, 277–284.

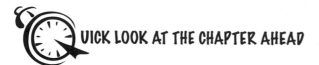

QUICK LOOK AT THE CHAPTER AHEAD

Patients with Human Deficiency Virus (HIV) commonly experience physical pain, which is often unrecognized and/or undertreated. Identification of the source of the pain is often challenging for healthcare providers, especially those unfamiliar with the complexities of HIV disease and its treatments. It is essential that providers be educated about common causes of pain in this patient population in order to recognize the pain, and facilitate appropriate evaluation and treatment.

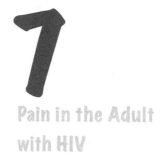

7

Pain in the Adult with HIV

TERMS
- ☐ antiretroviral agents
- ☐ antiretroviral therapy (ART)
- ☐ arthralgias
- ☐ candidiasis
- ☐ cytochrome P450 3A4 enzyme system
- ☐ didanosine
- ☐ efavirenz
- ☐ emtricitabine
- ☐ indinavir
- ☐ Kaposi's Sarcoma (KS)
- ☐ lamivudine
- ☐ myalgias
- ☐ peripheral neuropathy
- ☐ reflexology
- ☐ seropositive
- ☐ tenofovir
- ☐ vesicles
- ☐ zidovudine

117

CASE STUDY

T. D. is a 32-year-old female who has had human immunodeficiency virus (HIV) for 5 years. Over the past four years, T.D. has been on a variety of antiviral therapies, which included zidovudine (Retrovir®), didanosine (ddI), and indinavir (Crixivan®). She is currently taking **emtricitabine** (Emtriva®), **tenofovir** (Viread®), and **efavirenz** (Sustiva®).

Today T. D. presents to the clinic with recent onset of mouth pain but has no fever or dental problems. When asked about the presence of other symptoms of discomfort,

What was the likely cause of T.D.'s headaches last year? What did the burning and tingling in T. D.'s feet likely represent and what was the likely cause? What was the likely cause of T. D.'s muscle aches? What are possible causes of T. D.'s mouth pain?

she states she is having only a rare headache, as opposed to last year when she was having them frequently. She denies burning and tingling in her feet, which she had last year when she was taking ddI. She also states that the muscle aches in her legs occur less frequently and are less intense than previously.

PREVALENCE OF PAIN RELATED TO HIV INFECTION

Infection with HIV puts an individual at high risk for experiencing a variety of pain syndromes. Knowledge of the common symptoms and patterns of pain related to HIV infection assists providers in identifying the cause, significance, and treatment. Because pain can indicate a life-threatening infection, malignancy, or reaction to a drug, each new pain should be recognized as potentially significant and, if necessary, the client should be referred to an infectious disease specialist with expertise in HIV.

Statistics on the prevalence of pain in clients with HIV infection vary, but it is known that pain can occur at any point throughout the HIV trajectory. A study reported in 1993 found that 53 (28%) of 191 **seropositive** men with asymptomatic disease had HIV-related pain. According to one study in 1998, 40% to 60% of clients with HIV had pain.

Studies of clients with acquired immunodeficiency syndrome (AIDS) indicate that pain is present in 50% to 80%, and that it is more severe than during earlier stages. Pain related to HIV is often compared to pain related to cancer in terms of its prevalence, intensity, impact on quality of life, treatment, and undertreatment. Intensity of the pain also increases with progression of HIV, as it does with cancer. The client with HIV commonly has two to three sources of pain at a time, whereas the client with cancer has an average of three. As seen in clients with cancer, pain in clients with HIV also has a negative impact on an individual's quality of life. It can lead to functional disabilities, social isolation, depression, hopelessness, and suicidal ideation. Comprehensive assessment of the physiological, psychological, sociocultural, developmental, and spiritual dimensions of a client's life is necessary to adequately address the pain and its impact.

 # ETIOLOGIES OF PAIN RELATED TO HIV INFECTION

Assessing for the etiology of pain in clients with HIV is particularly challenging because opportunistic diseases, malignancies, and treatments cause pain in so many systems of the body, and the cause of each pain is not always identifiable.

Pain associated with HIV can be related to:

1. An opportunistic infection/condition or malignancy secondary to HIV
2. The virus itself
3. Medication given as treatment of the virus
4. Pathology unrelated to HIV

In terms of duration, HIV-related pain may be acute or chronic. Acute or short-term pain is directly related to tissue injury and resolves with tissue healing. An example of short-term pain related to an opportunistic condition is pain in the oropharynx due to inflammation from **candidiasis** overgrowth. An example of short-term pain related to treatment for HIV is abdominal pain associated with acute pancreatitis, which is a side effect of certain antiretroviral agents such as **didanosine (ddI)** and **lamivudine** (Epivir).

Chronic pain can occur due to HIV pathology (that is, damage to tissue caused by the virus itself), infections, malignancies, or as a side effect of medications such as antiretrovirals. Chronic pain may be persistent or episodic, and it is classified as somatosensory, visceral, or neuropathic. Somatosensory pain arises from bones, muscles, joints, or skin, and is often described as sharp, aching, or throbbing. Visceral pain originates from organ capsules, and varies with the structures involved. It is generally more diffuse in its location. Obstruction of a hollow viscous is associated with cramping or gnawing pain. Injury to other visceral organs is characterized by aching, stabbing, or throbbing pain. Although it is commonly associated with organs in the abdominal cavity, visceral pain can occur elsewhere, such as in the intrapleural space. Neuropathic pain originates from the central or peripheral nervous system, and is characterized as sharp, burning, shooting, shock-like, tingling, prickling, aching, an uncomfortable numbness, or a combination of the above. It frequently begins in the hands and the feet, but can also involve larger nerves in the chest or other areas of the body. At times, neuropathic pain is difficult for the patient to localize.

 # COMMON SYNDROMES OF PAIN WITH HIV INFECTION

Common syndromes of pain related to HIV include headache, **arthralgias**, **myalgias**, painful **peripheral neuropathy**, pharyngeal pain, abdominal pain, painful dermatological conditions, and pain due to extensive **Kaposi's sarcoma (KS)**.

Headaches

Headaches are prevalent in HIV-infected patients, and they occur more frequently in women. HIV-related headaches could be caused by infections such as bacterial sinusitis, cryptococcal meningitis, or toxoplasmosis encephalitis; malignancies such as lymphoma; or medications such as **zidovudine**, didanosine, or **indinavir**. Headaches may also be an exacerbation of a pre-existing migraine or tension headache syndrome.

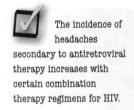 The incidence of headaches secondary to antiretroviral therapy increases with certain combination therapy regimens for HIV.

New onset or increased intensity of a headache should be evaluated promptly by a healthcare provider to rule out a life-threatening cause. Life-threatening disorders that present with a headache include meningitis and lymphoma.

One clinical trial of 196 clients compared the use of zidovudine, zidovudine combined with indinavir, and indinavir alone. The incidence of headaches increased from 5.6% to 11.7% when both zidovudine and indinavir were taken. The same study showed that the incidence of headaches decreased to 5.1% when indinavir was taken alone. A clinical trial of 230 clients taking zidovudine and lamivudine found that the incidence of headaches increased from 27% in clients taking zidovudine alone to 35% in those taking these drugs together.

Treatment of headaches involves treating the underlying cause and providing symptomatic support. Individuals with headaches secondary to **antiretroviral therapy (ART)** should have their medication regimen evaluated by physicians and nurses who are experienced with these drugs to evaluate the benefits of the therapy given the adverse effects, and consider trying medication regimens less likely to cause headaches.

Patients experiencing headaches secondary to ART should be provided with analgesics, the potency of which is based on the severity and the frequency of the pain. Acetaminophen on an as-needed basis may be sufficient for headaches of mild intensity. A more potent medication such as oxycodone or oxycodone acetaminophen combination (for example, Percocet, Tylox) should be offered for headaches of moderate to severe intensity. Patients who do not obtain adequate

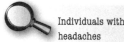 Individuals with headaches secondary to ART should have their medication regimen monitored by physicians and nurses experienced with these drugs to evaluate the benefits of the therapy given the adverse effects.

relief from this or any other medication should be evaluated for change to another narcotic. Changes in antiretroviral regimens also depend on each client's tolerance to side effects and ability to adhere to treatment plans.

Clients with HIV-related headaches might also benefit from nonpharmacological interventions used in conjunction with medications. Resting in a dark, quiet environment with a cold washcloth or ice bag placed on the forehead could facilitate relief. Frontal headaches secondary to sinus congestion may improve with warmth and steam. Headaches originating at the back of the head or neck often represent muscle tension as a source. Heat and massage, acupressure, and **reflexology** (massage limited to the feet or hands) can be effective for muscle tension.

Pharyngeal Pain

Pharyngeal pain that causes difficulty swallowing is usually related to fungal overgrowth (commonly *Candida*), herpes simplex, or KS. Other causes include ulcerative lesions of infectious or nonspecific origins. Treatment of pharyngeal pain involves treating the underlying cause and providing symptomatic support. Local or systemic antifungal agents are prescribed for infections suspected to be fungal. Acyclovir is prescribed if the lesions appear like **vesicles** (for example, herpetic lesions).

Candida stomatitis, which is a frequent finding with AIDS, often progresses to the esophagus, which can cause retrosternal pain (behind the ribs). Women with HIV or AIDS also may have pain secondary to vaginal candidiasis.

Muscle and Joint Pain

Myalgia refers to pain in muscle, and arthralgia refers to pain in a joint. Several arthritis and arthralgia syndromes related to HIV infection and HIV-related illnesses are known to cause chronic somatic pain in joints, muscles, and other tissues. Examples of these syndromes include HIV-associated arthritis, nonspecific arthralgias, Reiter's syndrome, and psoriatic arthritis. Aseptic myositis and HIV-associated myositis can also occur. Arthralgias and myalgias that cause chronic somatic pain also occur as a side effect of antiviral drugs such as zidovudine. Myopathy characterized by muscle weakness, elevated creatinine kinase, myalgia, and cramping can occur secondary to HIV infection, microsporidia, zidovudine, isoniazid (INH), alcohol, or illicit drugs.

Nonsteroidal anti-inflammatory drugs (NSAIDs) may reduce inflammation and decrease discomfort associated with arthralgia and myalgia, without causing sedation.

Peripheral Neuropathy

Forty to 50% of patients infected with HIV experience some degree of painful neuropathy, with the severity and course of the pain varying greatly (**Table 7-1**). A generalized neuropathy may be caused by the virus itself; by HIV-related illnesses such as cytomegalovirus, herpes zoster, or mycobacterium; or by medications, alcohol, or vitamin deficiencies

Table 7-1 Causes of Peripheral Neuropathy

Human immunodeficiency virus	
Select antiretrovial agents	Didanosine (ddI, Videx)
	Stavudine (d4T, Zerit)
	Zalcitabine (ddc, HIVID)
	Lamivudine (Epivir, 3TC)
	Emtricitabine (Emtriva)
Conditions associated with HIV	Cytomegalovirus
	Herpes zoster
	Mycobacterium
Vitamin deficiencies (B$_6$, B$_{12}$)	
Select anti-infective agents	Metronidazole (Flagyl)
	Isoniazid
	Rifampin
	Ethionamide
Medications to treat cytomegalovirus	Foscarnet
Medications to prevent *Pneumocystis carinii* pneumonia	Dapsone
Medications to treat KS	Vincristine
	Vinblastine
Conditions unrelated to HIV	Diabetes
	Alcohol Use
	Immune-mediated inflammatory demyelination
	Mononeuritis multiplex

(for example, B$_6$, B$_{12}$). Medications used in treatment of HIV that cause peripheral neuropathy include certain **antiretroviral agents** (for example, didanosine, lamivudine, stavudine, zalcitabine), certain anti-infective agents (for example, metronidazole, isoniazid, rifampin, ethionamide), medications to treat cytomegalovirus (for example foscarnet), medications to prevent *Pneumocystis carinii* pneumonia (for example dapsone), and medications to treat KS (for example vincristine, vinblastine). If the cause of the peripheral neuropathy is thought to be a medication, the dose of the medication is decreased or the drug may be stopped.

Conditions unrelated to HIV that can cause peripheral neuropathy include diabetes, immune-mediated inflammatory demyelination, and mononeuritis multiplex.

Certain types of ART, the mainstay of treatment for HIV infection, often cause painful syndromes such as peripheral neuropathy.

Tricyclic antidepressants, such as amitriptyline (Elavil®) are the drugs of choice to treat peripheral neuropathy, but individuals with HIV infection can be very sensitive to them. Anticonvulsants such as carbamazepine (Tegretol®) and lamotrigine (Lamictal®) are also effective in relieving neuropathic pain, but their levels need to be monitored. Opioids are given to treat peripheral neuropathic pain, especially while waiting for antidepressants or anticonvulsant therapy to be effective.

Because adherence to antiretroviral schedules is vital to optimal treatment for HIV infection, clients need to be monitored closely for their tolerance and willingness to take ART.

Abdominal Pain

Abdominal pain in a client with HIV infection can be caused by acute or chronic gastrointestinal infections with *Campylobacter*, *Shigella*, *Salmonella*, *Cryptosporidiosis*, cytomegalovirus, or *Mycobacterium intracellulare*. Abdominal pain can also be caused by pancreatitis associated with ART, pentamidine, or cytomegalovirus. Organomegaly, secondary to tumor invasion of organs with lymphoma or KS, is also a cause.

Dermatological Pain

Clients with KS can experience severe pain due to direct infiltration of the tumors into the skin or to associated lymphedema. Treatment of pain includes narcotic analgesics, and it may include chemotherapy to treat KS. However, both vincristine and vinblastine, which are used to treat KS, are potential causes of peripheral neuropathy.

ANALGESICS FOR HIV-RELATED PAIN

Treatment of pain related to HIV infection should be aimed at treating the cause. However, treatment of the cause does not always alleviate the pain, and identification of the cause is not always possible. Adequate treatment of HIV-related pain frequently requires the use of pharmacological agents on either a short- or long-term basis. Treatment for HIV-related pain should be fundamentally the same as the treatment of cancer pain, and it should be guided by standardized clinical practice guidelines such as those published on the Management of Cancer Pain by the Agency for Healthcare Policy and Research (AHCPR) (Jacox et al., 1994). These guidelines promote use of the World Health Organization (WHO) analgesic ladder, which bases treatment on the severity of the pain. Nonopioid analgesics should be used for mild pain, and opioid analgesics for moderate to severe pain. Morphine sulfate is considered the drug of choice for moderate to severe pain, with the oral route and controlled-release medications being the most widely used. Adjuvant medications should be used in addition to an opioid for neuropathic pain. Other principles of pain management that guide treatment of HIV-related pain include recommendations to give around-the-clock medications to prevent chronic pain and short-acting analgesics for breakthrough pain. AHPCR guidelines on pain also recommend the use of equianalgesic conversions, use of a variety of interventions to control pain (for example, complementary therapies such as massage, imagery, therapeutic touch) and comprehensive assessments and treatments that address the multidimensional aspects of the person (physiological, psychosocial, spiritual, and developmental).

The inability to identify a definitive cause of pain in a patient with HIV should not hinder healthcare providers from prescribing effective analgesics for the patient's pain.

Physicians specializing in infectious disease who are knowledgeable about the complexities of HIV disease and HIV treatment should be consulted for painful syndromes of unknown causes. Infectious disease experts are more apt to have in-depth, up-to-date knowledge of the illness and its ever-evolving treatment.

Updated information on pain management in individuals with HIV can also be obtained from the American Pain Society's *Principles of Analgesic Use in the Treatment of Acute Pain and Cancer Pain*. Of particular significance is the fact that antiretrovirals such as ritonavir and indinavir inhibit the **cytochrome P450 3A4 enzyme system** in the liver, which metabolizes methadone, hydrocodone, fentanyl, and oxycodone. Medications that inhibit this enzyme system can slow the metabolism of these opioids, and cause a higher peak effect and longer duration of opioid action, increasing the risk of adverse effects such as sedation or respiratory depression.

COMPLEMENTARY THERAPIES FOR HIV-RELATED PAIN

Regardless of the cause, clients with pain often benefit from the practice of complementary therapies used in conjunction with pharmacological interventions. Clients with HIV are no exception to this rule. In fact, surveys indicate that up to 70% of clients infected with HIV have sought some form of alternative or complementary therapy. Complementary therapies are particularly appropriate for use in this client population because of their enhancing effect on the immune system and their low risk for adverse effects. Examples of complementary therapies shown to alleviate pain in clients with HIV include chiropractic, osteopathic, and massage therapies for musculoskeletal symptoms and peripheral neuropathies, and therapeutic touch for peripheral neuropathies and other HIV-associated pain.

CASE STUDY RESOLVED

Headaches in a patient with HIV infection may be related to a central nervous system infection or malignancy. Once these causes are ruled out, ART is often considered to be the cause. Headaches are often a side effect of taking zidovudine and/or indinivir. T. D. was taking zidovudine and indinavir when she had headaches last year. Peripheral neuropathy occurs secondary to the antiretroviral drug ddI, which T. D. was taking when she had the burning and tingling in her feet. The burning and tingling resolved after she stopped taking ddI. Somatic pain such as muscle aches often occurs in HIV-infected individuals. It may be associated with nonspecific arthralgias or myalgias, or may occur as a side effect of zidovudine. The fact that T. D.'s muscle pain has decreased may be an effect of discontinuing the zidovudine, or may be indicative of better control of the HIV infection. A decrease in viral load would support this. Finally, causes of mouth pain in a person with HIV infection include fungal overgrowth, herpes simplex, and KS.

Knowledge of patterns of HIV-related pain in conjunction with T. D.'s known HIV infection alerts the healthcare provider to T. D.'s report of mouth pain, headaches, and leg pain. Additional information about the location, character, intensity, and treatment of her headaches and leg pain is obtained, and a targeted physical assessment of her oral cavity and neurological system is performed. Findings of this assessment are evaluated in view of her current medications and past history.

Assessment of the oral cavity reveals creamy, white plaques on the tongue and buccal mucosa. Based on her history of oral candidiasis, the healthcare provider believes that recurrent oral candidiasis is responsible for T.D.'s mouth pain. Treatment of the cause of the pain (the candidiasis) with Nystatin suspension, lozenges, or other antifungal medications should relieve the oral pain as the candida overgrowth clears. The goal of treatment for candidiasis is complete resolution of the lesions and pain. It is important that T.D. be able to tolerate a full course of treatment to achieve complete resolution. Dislike for the taste of an antifungal suspension could risk nonadherence and incomplete response. The healthcare provider assesses the client's willingness to follow through with liquid antifungal treatment and offers an antifungal agent in pill form if that will facilitate adherence. It should be noted, however, that antifungal agents have multiple drug interactions, and caution needs to be used in prescribing them to people with HIV. For example, efavirenz levels are increased by the antifungal agent ketoconazole. Therefore, ketoconazole would not be the antifungal agent of choice for T.D.

The fact that T.D. has no further burning and tingling in her feet suggests that this pain (which she had last year) represented peripheral neuropathy, likely caused by ddI. When T. D. experienced this in the past, she admitted that she stopped taking her ddI because she could not tolerate the pain. T.D.'s pain and inability to follow a medication regimen with ddI prompted the change in ART to a regimen with less risk for neuropathy and nonadherence to the medication schedule. Once T.D. stopped taking the ddI and indinivir, the peripheral neuropathy resolved, and she followed the new antiviral regimen. Healthcare providers should continue to assess T.D. for neuropathy-type pain, however, which could occur as an adverse effect of emtricitabine (Emtriva).

T.D.'s report of only rare headaches (as opposed to frequent) is likely an outcome of discontinuing the zidovudine and indinavir. If she had a headache of new onset that was associated with fever, or had an increase in frequency and intensity of headaches, it would be a significant concern. It should be noted that headaches are a common adverse effect of the ART emtricitabine (Emtriva), which T.D. is currently taking. T.D. states that she takes two tablets of acetaminophen to relieve her rare headache, with good effect.

The fact that T.D.'s muscle pain in her legs has decreased in frequency likely represents either the effect of discontinuing zidovudine or better control of the HIV itself. A decrease in the measurement of T. D.'s viral load would support improved control of HIV.

Discussion of T.D.'s pain would not be complete without mention of the potential effect pain has on the psychosocial and other dimensions of life, and the effect that these dimensions have on her pain. It is important to recognize that pain in women with HIV infection is twice as likely to be undertreated than pain in men, and that pain in patients with HIV infection and a history of drug abuse is 1.8 times as likely to be undertreated. Although nurses do not prescribe analgesics, they play a major role in the treatment of pain. Nurses advocating for clients with pain should understand that injustices in the treatment of pain based on gender and histories of drug abuse exist and interfere with effective treatment and quality of life. Studies looking at the use of analgesia for HIV-related pain indicate that patients with histories of drug abuse do not use more analgesics than those without histories of drug abuse. Nurses and healthcare providers should not be distracted with concerns about possible abuse of analgesics in this patient population. They should, instead, focus their efforts on relieving the patient's pain.

If an effective analgesia for HIV-related pain is chosen, clients will achieve relief of pain 75% to 80% of the time. In some patients, the source of pain is not identifiable, despite a comprehensive work-up. The inability to identify the source of pain in a client with HIV is not uncommon, and it is an inappropriate reason for withholding pain medication. The potential and actual effects of inadequate treatment of pain on the client's quality of life should guide the treatment of pain, regardless of the cause or the circumstances.

CHAPTER 7 · REVIEW QUESTIONS

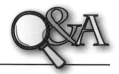

1. In clients with HIV, headaches of moderate intensity that are not relieved by acetaminophen should be treated with:
    A. Aspirin
    B. Ibuprofen
    C. Morphine
    D. Oxycodone

2. Recommended nonpharmacological interventions for headaches related to HIV:
    A. Are not as effective as medications
    B. Are more effective than medications
    C. Should be used in conjunction with medications
    D. Should not be used in conjunction with antiretrovirals

3. Antiretrovirals that are most often responsible for pain-related peripheral neuropathy include:
    A. Didanosine (ddI), zalcitabine (ddC), and stavudine
    B. Indinovir and ddI
    C. Lamiduvine and indinovir
    D. Zidovudine and lamiduvine

4. The class of medications that is considered the preferred treatment for painful peripheral neuropathy in clients with HIV is:
    A. Antiretrovirals
    B. Protease inhibitors
    C. Tricyclic antidepressants
    D. Nonsteroidal anti-inflammatory drugs (NSAIDs)

5. A "new" symptom of pain in a client with HIV should be:
    A. Fully assessed and reported to the physician
    B. Monitored while withholding treatment
    C. Treated with analgesics
    D. Treated with complementary therapies

ANSWERS AND RATIONALES

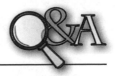

1. **D.** Acetaminophen on an as-needed basis may be sufficient for headaches of mild intensity. A more potent medication such as oxycodone or a combination of oxycodone and acetaminophen should be offered for headaches of moderate to severe intensity.

2. **C.** Heat, cold, massage, acupressure, and reflexology have been recommended for use in conjunction with medication.

3. **A.** Certain antiretrovirals used in the treatment of HIV cause peripheral neuropathy. These include ddI, ddC, and stavudine.

4. **C.** Opioids may be used to treat pain related to peripheral neuropathy, but tricyclic antidepressants are the drugs of choice.

5. **A.** New symptoms of pain in clients with HIV must be promptly assessed to rule in or rule out the cause. This is particularly important because an infectious etiology can be life threatening. Initiation of appropriate treatment may be essential to keeping the client alive or maintaining quality of life.

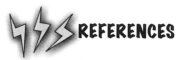

REFERENCES

American Pain Society. (2003). *Principles of analgesic use in the treatment of acute pain and cancer pain* (5th. ed). Glenview, IL: Author.

Breitbart, W. (1996). Pharmacotherapy of pain in AIDS. In G. P. Wormser (Ed), *A clinical guide to AIDS and HIV* (pp. 359–378). Philadelphia: Lippincott-Raven.

Breitbart, W. (1998). *Pain management in HIV/AIDS.* Paper presented at the 9th National Meeting for State Cancer Pain Initiatives, Portland, ME.

Breitbart, W., Rosenfeld, B. D., Passik, S. D., McDonald, M. V., Thaler, H., & Portenoy, R. (1996). The undertreatment of pain in ambulatory AIDS patients. *Pain, 65*(2/3), 243–249.

Cabaleiro, J. (2002). Assessing and treating neuropathic pain. *Home Healthcare Nurse, 20*(11), 718–723.

Elliott, J., Knox, K., Renaud, E., et al. (2002). Chronic pain management. In B. St. Marie (Ed.), *Core curriculum for pain management nursing* (pp. 273–347). Philadelphia: W.B. Saunders.

Jacox, A., Carr, D. B., Payne, R., et al. (1994). *Management of cancer pain. Clinical practice guideline No. 9. AHCPR Pub. No. 94-0592.* Rockville, MD: U.S. Public Health Service, AHCPR.

O'Neill, J. F., Selwyn, P. A., & Schietinger, H. (Eds.). (2003). *A clinical guide to supportive and palliative care for HIV/AIDS.* Washington, DC: Health Resources and Services Administration.

Palliative care model lost in today's HIV/AIDS care. (2006). *AIDS Alert, 21*(11), 129–131.

Portenoy, R. K. (1997). *Pain in oncologic and AIDS patients.* Newtown, PA: Handbooks in Health Care.

Sampson, J. G. (2006). Interventions for clients with HIV/AIDS and other immunodeficiencies. In D. Ignatavicius & M. L. Workman (Eds.), *Medical-surgical nursing* (5th ed., pp. 423–452). St. Louis, MO: Elsevier Saunders.

Singer, E., Surlier, C., Fahy-Chandon, B., Chi, S., Syndulko, K., & Tourtellotte, W. (1993). Painful symptoms reported by HIV-infected men in a longitudinal study. *Pain, 54*, 15–19.

Wentz, J. (2005). Managing pain in a patient with HIV or AIDS. *Nursing, 35*(6), 28.

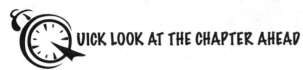

A specific cause for low back pain is often difficult to diagnose, and therefore difficult to treat. Low back pain that lingers and develops into chronic pain can negatively impact all aspects of a person's life, leading to depression and even suicide. Because primary care providers are often not skilled in providing effective treatment for chronic pain, it is imperative that they refer clients with unrelieved back pain to specialists knowledgeable in effective therapies.

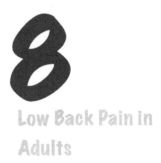

8

Low Back Pain in Adults

TERMS
- [ ] ankylosing spondylitis
- [ ] annular tears
- [ ] cyclobenzaprine
- [ ] degenerative disc disease
- [ ] disc herniation
- [ ] facet syndrome
- [ ] lumbosacral sprain
- [ ] lumbosacral strain
- [ ] myofascial
- [ ] physiatrist
- [ ] spondylolisthesis
- [ ] spondylopathy
- [ ] spondylosis
- [ ] spondylolysis
- [ ] zygapophyseal joints

CASE STUDY

Mrs. K. is a 30-year-old woman who works as a registered nurse in a community hospital. While caring for a patient in cardiac arrest, she injures her lower back. Mrs. K. is examined by an orthopedic surgeon, who finds no neurological deficits and no significant abnormalities on radiographic study of the spine. A diagnosis of lumbosacral strain is made, and Mrs. K. is provided with a plan of care consisting of bed rest for 3 days, ibuprofen 400 mg every 6 hours, **cyclobenzaprine** (Flexeril®) 10 mg three times a day, and moist heat as needed. She is also instructed not to return to work or perform strenuous activity (for example, lifting) until she has been cleared by the physician.

For more than 1 week, Mrs. K. remains on bed rest, walking to the bathroom as needed. Her pain initially improves with rest, so she continues to limit her activity as much as possible. She states she is afraid that any increase in her activity will cause **disc herniation**. She stops taking her cyclobenzaprine but increases the dose of ibuprofen to 600 mg every 6 hours.

On follow-up visits with her physician 4 and 8 weeks after injury, she informs the physician that her pain continues, and that she has new pain in her buttocks. He tells her that there is no evidence of a disc disorder and that she can return to work for 4-hour periods. There is no discussion about her pain experience, and no other recommendations for treatment or symptom relief are made.

When Mrs. K. returns to work, she finds that she is extremely stiff, with dull pain in her low back after 4 hours. After several days of work, much of her stiffness is relieved, but her pain continues. Ten weeks after injury, the orthopedic surgeon tells her she may return to work full-time and releases her from his care. Out of frustration, Mrs. K. makes an appointment with her primary care physician, who tells her there is nothing wrong neurologically and gives her a handout with instructions for pelvic tilt exercises. Mrs. K. performs the exercises as prescribed by the physician but finds that they do not help relieve the pain. Frustrated and concerned that she may not be performing the exercises properly, she refers herself to a physical therapist who is described as someone with expertise in back pain. The therapist urges Mrs. K. to increase the number of pelvic tilts she is doing and gives her additional exercises to strengthen her back.

Mrs. K. finds that one of the exercises (upper trunk extension) helps relieve her pain, but that the pelvic tilt (a flexion exercise) actually increases the pain intensity. Because she is concerned she will harm herself further, Mrs. K. stops doing the pelvic tilts. On sharing this information with the therapist, the therapist tells Mrs. K. that there is nothing more she can do for her if she is not going to do her exercises.

Concerned that she is not improving, Mrs. K. again contacts her primary care physician to request a computed tomography (CT scan). Before this is ordered, she is required to see her physician, who reassesses her neurological status and finds no deficits. The physician agrees to order a CT scan,

 Identify three questions that Mrs. K. might have asked the orthopedic surgeon while he was caring for this client. Why do you think the orthopedic surgeon released Mrs. K. without ordering physical therapy and/or follow-up? Why do you think Mrs. K's primary care physician gave her no further recommendation for treatment of her back pain? Which characteristic of Mrs. K's pain support the diagnosis of myofascial pain?

which is performed 1 week later. Three weeks after the scan, the physician notifies Mrs. K. that the CT findings are normal. He gives her no further recommendations to help with her pain.

 ## TYPES OF LOW BACK PAIN

The causes of low back pain are many and varied. In a study evaluating the pathophysiology of back pain, 4% of patients had a compression fracture, 3% had **spondylolisthesis**, 0.7% had a tumor or metastasis, 0.3% had **ankylosing spondylitis**, and 0.01% had an infection. The most common cause of back pain was (and remains) nonspecific, and attributed to the degenerative process of the spine, known as **spondylosis**. Muscular and ligament inflammation are causes of low back pain in another large percentage of Americans.

The most common cause of back pain is nonspecific, and it is attributed to the degenerative process of the spine. Muscular and ligament inflammation cause low back pain in another large percentage of Americans.

Specific causes of low back pain are difficult to diagnose. Radiographic studies (x-rays) will show the bony anatomy of the spine, and can rule in or rule out fractures, tumors, and congenital abnormalities, but these are not the major causes of back pain. **Degenerative disc disease** is often seen on x-rays. However, simply finding evidence of this on x-ray does not explain back pain, because degenerative disease occurs in almost half the population, yet most of these people are asymptomatic. Diagnostic tests such as magnetic resonance imaging (MRI) are more valuable for diagnosing soft tissue, muscle, and ligament abnormalities. However, MRIs are not routinely performed on clients with acute low back pain. They are generally reserved for clients who have back pain lasting more than 1 month that does not respond to treatment.

 Degenerative disc disease is often seen on x-rays, but simply finding evidence of this on x-ray does not explain back pain because degenerative disease occurs in almost half the population, and most of these people are asymptomatic.

When diagnostic tests, physical examination findings, and the client's history rule in or rule out certain abnormalities, more specific diagnoses for low back pain can sometimes be made. Diagnostic labels (**Table 8-1**) for specific types of degenerative disc disease or muscular or ligamentous causes of low back pain include:

- lumbosacral strain or sprain
- disc herniation/herniated intervertebral disk
- discogenic syndrome
- **facet syndrome**
- spinal stenosis
- **spondylolysis**
- spondylolisthesis
- spondylosis

Because evidence to support one of these specific diagnoses is often lacking, low back pain is frequently described in terms of its duration (for example, acute versus chronic) and site (for example, lumbosacral spine), as opposed to its cause.

Acute Low Back Pain

Most occurrences of low back pain are acute, self-limiting, and benign, lasting less than 1 month. Some occurrences last longer, but most resolve within 3 months. Patients with low back pain should have a history and physical examination, with an emphasis on the severity of pain and

Table 8-1 Diagnostic Labels for Low Back Pain

Disc herniation: herniation or displacement of the nucleus pulposus partly or completely through a defect in the annulus from the intervertebral space into the spinal canal or foramen or outside the foramen.

Discogenic syndrome: imprecise term that suggests annulus tears and release of a chemical mediator from the lumbar disc, resulting in pain.

Facet syndrome: pain in the facets, also referred to as zygapophyseal joints; this pain is located only in the back and is aggravated by movement, particularly rotation, and improves with rest.

Lumbosacral strain or **sprain**: muscular and ligamentous injury.

Spinal stenosis: old term describing the condition when the spinal canal is narrowed either congenitally or from spondylosis.

Spinal instability: occurs when movement of bony elements is identified on flexion or extension, on motion films, or in repeated studies. The definition is controversial.

Spondylolysis: a structural defect in the pars interarticularis.

Spondylolisthesis: slipping of one vertebral segment onto another.

Spondylosis: general term that describes all the changes that occur with degenerative disc disease, including desiccation of the disc, narrowing of the interspace, inflammatory and degenerative changes in the bone, ligament hypertrophy, and bone spurring.

Spondylopathy: disease of the vertebrae

---

neurological function below the level of the pain. Severe pain or pain considered to be related to trauma, metastatic disease, or neurological dysfunction will likely prompt the physician to obtain x-rays of the spine, MRI, and a consultation with a back specialist. A CT scan may be of some value in diagnosing the source of pain, but CT scans are limited by the fact that they do not show soft tissue injury. MRI is often the test of choice because it not only shows soft tissue injury, but also shows disc herniation with great accuracy.

Unless pain is severe without alleviation after medication or rest, or related to significant trauma or a malignancy, imagery studies (that is, CT scan or MRI) are generally not required for acute back pain. Imaging studies are reasonable for back pain lasting 1 month or longer. However, they do not consistently identify the pathology.

Most causes of acute low back pain originate within muscles or ligaments of the back. Diagnostic labels related to acute low back pain include:

- lumbosacral strain or sprain
- disc herniation
- injury to **zygapophyseal joints**
- minor **annular tears**

A **lumbosacral strain** or **sprain** implies a muscle or ligament injury, similar to an ankle sprain. A diagnosis of **disc herniation** should be made only when the nucleus pulposus has been displaced (or herniates) partly or completely from the intervertebral space through a defect in the annulus into the spinal canal or foramen or outside the foramen (**Figure 8-1**). True disc herniation is actually a rare cause of back pain, but clients with herniated discs typically have had previous episodes of acute back pain. In contrast, **degenerated discs** are common.

The goals for patients with acute low back pain are: 1) acute management; 2) rehabilitation; and 3) prevention of further injury. Acute pain and inflammation should be managed with rest, ice, and medications such as anti-inflammatory drugs, analgesics, and muscle relaxants. Use of opioid analgesics for a few days may be required for some episodes of

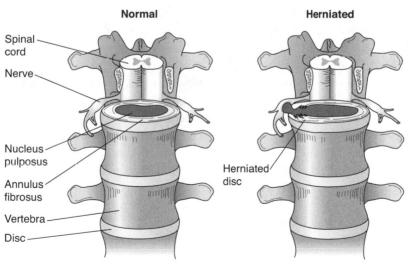

Figure 8-1   Herniated nucleus pulposus.

acute back pain. Patients with signs/symptoms of a herniated disc with neurologic changes (that is, decrease in motor function, deep tendon reflexes, or sensation) require immediate referral to an orthopedic surgeon or neurosurgeon.

Assessment by an expert in physical medicine and physical therapy is an important part of the treatment of acute pain in the rehabilitation phase and, if appropriate, the acute management phase. A comprehensive assessment will include analysis of the pain, functional ability of the patient, and information about patient needs, goals, and fears.

Most clients with acute low back pain are incapacitated no longer than 1 or 2 weeks. They benefit from returning to their previous level of activity as soon as it is tolerated. Identification of activities that aggravate the client's pain is important to assist the client in making modifications to daily routines to reduce the risk of aggravation of the injury. With recovery from pain, an exercise program is developed by the physical therapist and patient to help prevent recurrence.

Any client with back pain lasting 3 months or longer should have a full physical examination to rule in or out systemic causes (for example, malignancy).

Chronic Low Back Pain

Fifty to 80% of people with back pain will have a recurrence of their pain within one year, and 2 to 7% will develop chronic pain. Although there is no clear-cut point where acute back pain can be labeled chronic, the transition from acute to chronic most likely occurs before a period of 6 months. Persistent low back pain is now recognized as different, as pain associated with acute back pain diminishes and resolves. Persistent low back syndrome or chronic, benign pain involves similar processes as in acute pain, including nerve irritation, muscle spasm, and/or inflammation in the peripheral tissues and central nervous system (spinal cord and brain). Chronic pain, however, differs from acute pain in that it lacks the normal checks and balances that serve to dampen or modulate acute pain processes. The alterations in these checks and balances can also perpetuate the pain signal and are thought to be responsible for pain that occurs even after tissue heals.

Treatment of Chronic Low Back Pain

Because no one specific cause of back pain may be identified, treatment should be multidisciplinary and individualized. Chronic pain related to inflammation, muscles, or nerve involvement may be treated with anti-inflammatory medications, analgesics, and, if appropriate, anticonvulsants or antidepressants. All patients with chronic low back pain should also be assessed by an expert in physical medicine and/or a physical therapist with experience in treating back pain. Experts in physical medicine (for example, **physiatrists**) and physical therapists are uniquely qualified to develop plans for stretching, muscle conditioning, massage, exercise, heat or cold, electrical stimulation, and manipulation that will meet the individual needs of patients.

BARRIERS TO TREATMENT

Chronic back pain is one of the greatest problems in health care, and it often goes unrecognized for the devastating impact it can have on individuals, families, and the community at large. For the individual and family, it is the cause of a significant amount of physical and psychosocial pain and suffering, with debilitating, long-lasting effects. From the perspective of community, it puts an enormous financial burden on our healthcare system, which leads to increased insurance premiums and healthcare costs. Billions of dollars are spent each year on medical bills, and billions more are lost in wages for clients disabled by the pain.

In recent years, new, more effective treatments for individuals with chronic back pain have been identified. However, there are significant barriers to clients receiving effective treatment (**Table 8-2**). Many primary care physicians have not been taught about **myofascial** pain and treatment, and they are not familiar with the existence and effectiveness of programs for this and other types of back or muscle pain. The problem is compounded by the fact that most primary care providers have not been taught how to treat the person in pain holistically, particularly when the pain is chronic. Medical training for chronic pain has been almost nonexistent.

Even when referrals are made, there is risk that treatment for chronic back pain will not be provided. Treatment provided by pain specialists may not be fully paid by third-party payers. Limitation of reimbursable visits is

Table 8-2 Barriers to Effective Treatment of Chronic Back Pain

- Limited knowledge about the pathology
- Limited medical education on chronic benign back
- Limited options in Western medicine
- Lack of standardization in treatment
- Increase in pain over time
- Patient hopelessness

likely to occur when third-party payers perceive treatment as nonphysical in nature (that is, visits for instruction on behavioral strategies) or when treatment plans are not supported by a significant amount of research. Limited participation in treatment for chronic back pain runs the risk that the treatment will not be effective in providing relief.

Delays in referrals for appropriate treatment also pose barriers to the efficacy of treatment. Unrelieved severe pain changes the spine in such a way that prolongs and intensifies the pain experience. Treatment late in the pain cycle is often less effective than treatment nearer the onset. Over time, pain intensifies and deconditioning ensues, further intensifying the pain experience. Clients undergoing such negative experiences often lose hope that they will obtain relief of their pain. Loss of hope can lead to depression, which also intensifies the negativity of the experience and diminishes the overall quality of clients' lives.

CASE STUDY REVISITED

Mrs. K.'s experience with acute low back pain, which evolved into chronic back pain, exemplifies the significant deficits in the medical community's approach to this problem. The initial work-up (which ruled out a neurological deficit) was appropriate, as was the treatment plan for rest, anti-inflammatories, muscle relaxants, and heat. However, Mrs. K.'s continued bed rest and inactivity, with resulting "stiffness," and her fear that activity might cause neurological dysfunction indicated that she lacked knowledge about the importance of limited activity and stretching. Her inactivity and stiffness likely intensified her pain and acted as a barrier to her recovery.

The absence of a full assessment of Mrs. K.'s pain experience, her release from treatment despite the presence of ongoing pain, the absence of imaging studies after 12 weeks of back pain, and the lack of recommendations or referrals for evaluation by a physical therapist, provide further evidence that the plan of care was inadequate.

Appropriate treatment for Mrs. K. should have included assessments for the impact the pain had on her physical function, level of frustration and distress, and quality of life. Mrs. K. should also have been told that true herniations of discs are not very common and that some activity such as stretching would likely enhance her recovery, not put her in danger. She should have been referred to a pain specialist, or a physical therapist who is experienced in back pain, to assist with a structured plan of activity tailored to her individual needs. Interventions such as local ice applications and relaxation techniques would also have been appropriate. Mrs. K. may also have benefited from referral for therapeutic manipulation (adjustment) of the spine by a chiropractor or osteopath, particularly when her pain was acute. Research has shown that spinal manipulation is effective in relieving pain and improving physical function in a significant number of clients with acute low back pain. Some clients may benefit from spinal adjustments even for chronic pain.

 ## MYOFASCIAL PAIN

Twenty percent of chronic low back pain is related to myofascial pain. Myofascial pain is characteristically generalized, radiating to hips, buttocks, groin, and upper thighs. The radiation of pain, however, does not suggest or represent nerve root compression, such as that which occurs with herniation. The hallmark of myofascial pain is the discovery of specific areas of inflammation in the muscles, referred to as trigger points. Trigger points can often be palpated in deep muscle as small, hard, painful knots. These triggers are thought to occur either primary or secondary to prolonged muscle spasm. Common locations of trigger points related to low back pain involve the paravertebral muscles or the glutei and, less often, the thigh muscles and the area over the greater trochanter.

Treatment of myofascial pain involves local heat, massage, transcutaneous electrical nerve stimulation (TENS), and injections of saline, anesthetic, or a corticosteroid directly into the muscle. Injections may need to be repeated over days to weeks. Treatment of myofascial pain generally requires a physican specializing in physical medicine or in pain management. Once myofascial pain is controlled, clients should be guided through an exercise program to strengthen the involved muscles and avoid future pain.

CASE STUDY RESOLVED

Without physician referral, Mrs. K. seeks treatment with an osteopathic physician. This physician tells her that her pelvis and spine are out of alignment and performs an adjustment. She obtains relief from her pain for a few days at a time, but the pain reoccurs within a week or so after manipulation.

Hopeful that more can be done for her pain, Mrs. K. seeks a physician who specializes in back pain. In the phone book, she finds a back clinic affiliated with a community hospital and a clinic for sports injuries. She is given an appointment, which involves history and physical examination by a physiatrist who is also a pain specialist.

The physical examination performed by the physiatrist differs in that in addition to assessing her neurological function, he assesses for sites of pain (trigger points) by applying deep pressure to the muscles in the buttocks (glutei) and thigh. The physician identifies multiple trigger points in both buttocks and thighs, along with tenderness in the left lower part of the back. He tells her that she has myofascial pain syndrome and recommends that she have a course of physical therapy that includes ultrasonic massage to trigger points, manual trigger point massage, and gentle muscle stretching. He recommends that she initially see the physical therapist three times a week and that he will follow her progress closely. She has a follow-up appointment with the specialist in 3 weeks, at which time he injects her trigger points with normal saline solution.

With this combination of therapies, Mrs. K.'s pain decreases, and she is started on a physical exercise program to strengthen the involved muscles and improve her flexibility and physical function. Over a period of 5 months, the pain in Mrs. K.'s back, buttocks, and thighs significantly decreases to the point that it occurs only with certain activities. One activity that aggravates the pain is the performance of pelvic tilts. Although the physical therapist does not understand why this exercise aggravates her pain, she states that it is essential to listen to each individual person's body and suggests that she no longer perform pelvic tilts. The physician also encourages Mrs. K. to perform her own trigger point therapy by applying pressure to trigger sites when pain recurs.

Through self-referral to a physician who specializes in chronic back pain, Mrs. K. not only obtains relief of the pain but also learns to control her pain when it reoccurs, possibly preventing its reoccurrence through stretching and gentle exercises tailored to her specific needs.

When Mrs. K. reported the new pain in the buttocks (new location) 4 and 8 weeks post-injury and the continued low back pain to the orthopedic surgeon, his reply was that there was "not a disc problem." Mrs. K., however, would have benefited from knowing what the new buttock pain represented. It would also have been beneficial to find out what the surgeon thought was causing the pain (if not a disc), what the expected outcome was likely to be, and whether physical therapy or manipulation with a chiropractor might help or hurt.

Education in medical school has historically neglected the problem of muscle pain and the significance of myofascial trigger points and pain. If a physician has not been taught or does not recognize a myofascial trigger point problem, he or she will not order an appropriate consult or treatment. The primary care physician likely released Mrs. K. without further recommendations because he believed he had ruled out a serious problem by CT scan and a negative neurological exam. A CT scan, however, would not show soft tissue injury, and a negative neurological exam does not address the problem of myofascial pain. The primary care physician, like the orthopedic surgeon, did not have adequate knowledge of myofascial pain, and the diagnosis was not made.

Pain in Mrs. K's low back that radiated to the buttocks 8 weeks post injury was characteristic of this diagnosis. Myofascial pain often radiates to the hips, buttocks, groin, and upper thighs. The physiatrist's assessment of trigger points by applying deep pressure to the muscles in the buttocks (glutei) and thigh also characterized Mrs. K's pain as myofascial.

CHAPTER 8 • REVIEW QUESTIONS

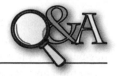

1. Specific causes of back pain are:
   A. Diagnosed through a medical history
   B. Diagnosed by x-ray
   C. Diagnosed by neurological exam
   D. Difficult to diagnose

2. Acute low back pain most often originates:
   A. In the bony portion of the spine
   B. In discs
   C. Within muscles or ligaments
   D. Within the spinal canal

3. The majority of clients with acute low back pain:
   A. Have herniated discs
   B. Develop chronic low back pain syndrome
   C. Are incapacitated no longer than 1 to 2 weeks
   D. Require surgery

4. Most clients with acute low back pain do not have neurological deficits. Recommended treatment for these clients includes all of the following EXCEPT:
   A. Bed rest for 1 week
   B. Anti-inflammatory drugs
   C. Analgesics
   D. Muscle relaxants

5. The hallmark of myofascial pain is:
   A. Improvement with bed rest
   B. Referred numbness and tingling
   C. A decrease in motor function
   D. Trigger points in muscles

ANSWERS AND RATIONALES

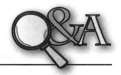

1. **D.** X-rays will show the bony anatomy of the spine, but soft tissue abnormalities are not well visualized. History and physical examination assist in ruling in and ruling out certain abnormalities but often do not give definitive information as to the specific cause of back pain.

2. **C.** Most causes of acute low back pain originate within muscles or ligaments of the back.

3. **C.** True disc herniation is actually a rare cause of back pain. Acute back pain is self-limiting and benign, and most clients are incapacitated no longer than 1 or 2 weeks. If neurological deficits are not involved, immediate surgery for back pain is generally not necessary.

4. **A.** Bed rest for clients with acute back pain should be limited to 3 days or less.

5. **D.** Trigger points are thought to occur either primary or secondary to prolonged muscle spasm.

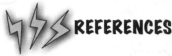

REFERENCES

Advise, H., Crombie, I., Brown, J., & Martin, C. (1997). Diminishing returns or appropriate treatment strategy? An analysis of short-term outcomes after pain clinic treatment. *Pain, 70*, 203–208.

Bigos, S., Bowyer, Q., Braen, G., et al. (1995). *Acute low back problems in adults: clinical practice guideline No. 14. AHCPR Pub No. 95-0643*. Rockville, MD: Agency for Health Care Policy and Research, Public Health Service, U.S. Department of Health and Human Services.

Caudill, M. (2001). *Managing pain before it manages you.* (2nd ed.). New York: Guilford Press.

Elliot, J., Knox, K., Renaud, E., St. Marie, B., Sharoff, L., Swift, M. K., et al. (2002). Chronic pain management (pp. 273–347). In B. St. Marie (Ed.), *Core curriculum for pain management nursing*. Philadelphia: W. B. Saunders.

Frymoyer, J. W. (1988). Back pain and sciatica. *N Engl J Med, 318*(5), 291–300.

Lavelle, W., Carl, A., & Lavelle, E. (2007). Invasive and minimally invasive surgical techniques for back pain conditions. In H. Smith (Ed.), *Medical clinics of North America pain management, part II 91*(2), 287–298.

Lavelle, E. D., Lavelle, W., & Smith, H. S. (2007). Myofascial trigger points. In H. Smith (Ed.), *Medical clinics of North America pain management, Part II 91*(2), 229–239.

Long, D. M. (1997).Contemporary diagnosis and management of pain. Newtown, PA: Handbooks in Health Care.

Travell, J. G., & Simons, D. G. (1983). Myofascial pain and dysfunction: the trigger point manual. Baltimore: Williams & Wilkins.

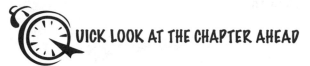
Specific considerations are part of pain management in children. To begin with, care of a child often includes care of the family unit as well. Communication issues and response patterns to adverse events make assessment for pain a challenge for the pediatric healthcare professional. Differences in both pharmacokinetics and pharmacodynamics add to the challenge of using medication safely. Considerations for developmental stages affect tactics for comfort, social support, and behavioral approaches to pain relief.

Pediatric clients are treated for pain across treatment settings, from home to outpatient ambulatory clinics, surgical and dental treatment centers, inpatient acute care facilities, long-term care facilities, and hospice. Acute pain is one of the most frequent reasons for accessing pediatric care. Strategies for pain control in this age group include pharmacological, physical, and behavioral options. All three options must be tailored to the age and developmental level of the child.

Historically, healthcare providers have had less success providing adequate interventions for pain in pediatric clients. By being aware of useful parameters at different stages of development, the healthcare provider can more expertly assess and plan interventions for pain.

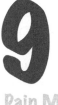

9

Pain Management in Children

TERMS

☐ absorption
☐ blood-brain barrier
☐ developmental stages
☐ distribution
☐ elimination
☐ family
☐ infants
☐ metabolism
☐ neonates
☐ pharmacokinetics
☐ preschool-age children
☐ regression
☐ toddlers

147

CASE STUDY

Brian B. is a 5-year-old boy who is admitted to the emergency room with a fractured left ulna. He is otherwise in good health. His father is with him, and they both appear very anxious. During the admission process, EMLA cream is applied to Brian's right forearm in preparation for intravenous (IV) access. The nurse anesthetist starts the IV with little discomfort to the client. As long as the fracture remains immobilized, Brian appears quite comfortable. A play therapist from the pediatrics department spends some time with Brian, helping him to stay occupied, relieve some of his stress, and reduce his exposure to the frightening environment of the emergency room. Finally, Brian is transported to have x-rays of the injury. As he has good color, sensation, and mobility above and below the fracture, it is determined by the radiologist that this simple fracture can be repaired though closed reduction in the emergency room.

 PAIN AND CHILDREN

Pediatric clients make up a group with very special needs when it comes to pain management. Communication issues and ways these clients respond to adverse events make assessment for pain different and more challenging. The challenge of using medication safely for pain control is presented because of the differences in uptake and metabolism. Varied **developmental stages** require varied approaches to comfort, social support, and behavioral approaches to pain relief. Including the parents in treatment decisions can be extremely important, but at the same time caregivers must not overwhelm them with information and tasks.

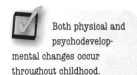
Both physical and psychodevelopmental changes occur throughout childhood.

 Children are not just small adults.

Developmental Considerations

Pediatric clients are usually grouped according to developmental stage. **Infants** are usually defined as birth to 1 year of age; children, 1 year through 11 years of age; and adolescents, 12 through 18 years of age. Children may be further grouped into toddlers, preschool-age children, and school-age children. All three groups have different levels of physical and psychosocial development, and differ-

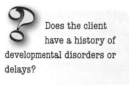

Does the client have a history of developmental disorders or delays?

ing developmental tasks. Both physical and psychosocial developmental stages should be considered when developing assessment and treatment plans for pain in the pediatric client. Elements at each stage of development affect how pain is perceived and relief measures that will be appropriate and helpful.

Although age is a good indicator of developmental stage in individual children, it is important to assess development rather than assume.

Common Types of Pain

The healthy child is more apt to experience acute forms of pain rather than chronic pain. Chronic pain is a factor in pediatric chronic illnesses or conditions and in congenital conditions. Acute pain may be the result of illness or occur with trauma, sur-

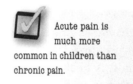

Acute pain is much more common in children than chronic pain.

gical intervention, or invasive diagnostic or treatment procedures. Pain in this client population is seen across treatment settings, from home to outpatient ambulatory settings, surgical and dental settings, inpatient acute care facilities, long-term care facilities, and hospice. Simple acute pain is one of the most frequent reasons for accessing pediatric care. This type of pain is often related to middle ear infection or swimmer's ear, teething pain, abdominal pain related to gastroenteritis or appendicitis, sore throat related to streptococcus infection or tonsillitis, or pain as the result of accidental trauma.

The Role of Parents in Assessment

The parent or adult caregiver is frequently the first one to identify the pain because of changes in the child's activity or demeanor. Depending on the changes noted and the adult's perceived severity of the pain or an assumption on the part of the adult as to the possible cause of the pain, independent measures for pain relief will be used or the child's healthcare provider will be called. Parents of young children who suffer frequent ear infections, for example, become expert at identifying pain-related behaviors such as changes in sleep and eating patterns, crying that is different from the norm, or self-comforting behaviors such as rubbing or tugging the affected ear. Experience builds a set of assessment parameters for these parents, and attention is more rapidly paid to these behaviors as indicating pain in the child.

 It is crucial to include the parent's input in assessment.

Intervention

Historically, pediatric clients have had less successful interventions for pain than adults. The reasons for this vary. The child's ability to express or communicate pain through behavior is often lacking and is sometimes

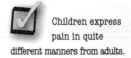 Children express pain in quite different manners from adults.

unrecognized. It is important to remember that a child is not a small adult. A healthcare provider cannot successfully provide interventions for what cannot be comprehensively assessed. To provide more successful intervention, better assessment tools and parameters must be identified for this population. Poor assessment impacts administration of analgesics or opioids when the medication is ordered on an as-needed (PRN) basis. Pain medication is often ordered to be given PRN, resulting in less effective pain relief for the often difficult-to-assess pediatric client. A PRN dosing schedule treats pain rather than attempting to keep the client relatively pain-free.

Many healthcare providers are reluctant to use opioids in the pain-relief plan for pediatric clients, choosing to use less potent analgesics. Even when opioids have been ordered, many nurses hesitate to choose them on a PRN basis, administering an ordered NSAID instead. As described in the Department of Health and Human Services pain management guidelines, when opioids are used, the dose is usually small, potentially inadequate to relieve pain, and time between doses is long, further hindering pain relief. This may relate to a caregiver's reluctance to use opioids or inability to effectively assess subtle cues indicating the presence of pain in the pediatric client. Adding to this problem is the current trend to order pain medication on a PRN basis. When subtle cues are missed in the assessment process, pain increases in severity before medication is offered for relief. Parents are included in the assessment process but are sometimes not believed. The first step to formulating a plan for adequate pain management in children as with all others is adequate, appropriate, and thorough assessment.

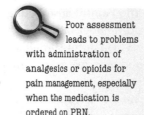 Poor assessment leads to problems with administration of analgesics or opioids for pain management, especially when the medication is ordered on PRN.

 A PRN dosing schedule treats pain rather than attempts to keep the client relatively pain-free

ASSESSING THE PEDIATRIC CLIENT FOR PAIN

How is it appropriate to assess the child for pain? What parameters are used? Children at different developmental stages react differently to pain. Reactions do not always seem to match severity. By being aware of useful parameters at different stages of development, the healthcare provider can more expertly assess and plan intervention.

 Parents of young children build their own assessment criteria. A parent is very often accurate in describing his or her young child's pain.

Developmental Strategies

Infants

Neonates (very young infants) cry as a result of pain. The intensity of the cry and associated vital signs may not indicate the intensity of the pain sensation. The cry may be weak, and heart rate and blood pressure may decrease instead of increasing.

As infants mature, crying continues to be the response to pain. Parents can often identify a distinctive cry related to pain that is different from other crying. Body movements will also change to indicate pain, including squirming, restlessness, and tugging

 Restlessness, changes in activity, crying behaviors and vital signs are all indicators of pain in infants.

at the painful area. Young infants will cry loudly and hold their bodies rigidly. Older infants react more specifically to pain, attempting to push away a painful stimulus. At this developmental point, heart rate and blood pressure are commonly elevated with pain. The older infant with a history of pain, especially painful procedures, may withdraw. Assessment in infants should include behavioral signs, like crying, and more subtle signs of pain, including body postures and vital signs.

Toddlers

Toddlers are more readily able to begin to engage in verbal communication but are still unable to talk about their pain. Physiological response to pain is similar to that of infants—loud, lusty crying and physical efforts to avoid painful stimulus. Toddlers in pain can be restless, even appearing hyperactive, even when increased activity exacerbates pain. This occurs because the toddler does not cognitively associate increased activity with increased pain. It is very important to be aware of this fact, because many adult caregivers tend to associate increasing levels of activity with feeling better. This is not necessarily so with the toddler. Expressions of pain continue to vary at this stage and with varied and emerging personality traits of each individual child, as well as increasing ability to communicate verbally.

Preschool-age Children

Preschool-age children are more developed in their verbal abilities, perceive the world in a very concrete and fixed way, have grave concerns about bodily mutilation, and can engage in magical thinking. These factors make assessment for pain very different from the younger child. Enhanced verbal abilities allow the preschooler to describe location and intensity of pain. Simple assessment scales are useful at this age, but scales involving numbers or printed words can be confusing or distracting. Intensity of color on a linear chart may be useful or the common happy to sad faces assessment tool (see Figure 2-5 in Chapter 2).

> A bandage to cover an injection site or injury is an important treatment for the magical thinking seen in this developmental group.

Verbal description scales such as "no pain, a little pain, a lot of pain, the worst pain" can be useful in evaluation of treatment, but it is important to keep the wording consistent. The

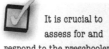

> It is crucial to assess for and respond to the preschooler's sense of self-blame or fear.

preschool-age child's reaction to pain may seem out of proportion with the event or the child's description of the pain. Fears, magical thinking, or a sense of self-blame may complicate this reaction. This child may also lash out angrily at caregivers, especially those involved in invasive procedures.

 Maintain consistency when caring for a preschooler.

School-age Children

School-age children have much improved powers of communication. They learn quickly, assimilating information, but giving it their own individual meaning. Thinking is very concrete. At this stage, the child can verbally describe location, intensity, and type or characteristics of pain, and can use most pain assessment scales. Avoid the temptation to treat this age group as a small adult. They are more passive than younger children about accepting pain and are much less able to verbalize requests for assistance or relief than the adult client.

 The child's stage of physical and psychosocial development directly affects pain perception, expression, and intervention.

Adolescents

Adolescents are even more developed in their ability to communicate but are frequently reluctant to communicate. Although they are well able to use assessment tools, their reluctance in communication requires the healthcare provider to assess for more subtle signs of pain. These include psychosocial withdrawal, decreased levels of activity, increased anger, suspicion, anxiety, or increased complaints about issues unrelated to pain. Vital signs such as blood pressure and heart rate generally increase with pain in this age group. Issues with sexuality and developing body image add to the adolescent's reluctance to express pain.

 Assessment and treatment of adolescents requires privacy and confidentiality.

Regression

It is not uncommon for a pediatric client to regress to thinking and behaviors that express pain in a younger developmental age group. The school-age child may act more like a pre-schooler or even a toddler. The toddler may only cry, not using developed verbal skills at all. Children who have recently achieved a developmental milestone, such as sentence construction or toilet training, may revert to old habits in the presence of pain. The preceding descriptions are useful as cues to assessment, but each individual pediatric client must be approached with assessment techniques that are appropriate for that individual.

 Are the behaviors observed normal for this individual, or the result of **regression** to an earlier developmental stage?

⚡⚡⚡ PAIN MANAGEMENT STRATEGIES FOR THE PEDIATRIC CLIENT

Strategies for pain control in this age group include pharmacological, physical, and behavioral options. All three options must be tailored to the age and developmental level of the child.

Pharmacological Interventions

Children use and metabolize medications in very different ways than adults. The safe and routine pediatric doses of medications are different from those of adults. Pharmacokinetics differs in children, especially in the infant and neonate. Pediatric healthcare providers must develop an understanding for these differences. In addition, it is the

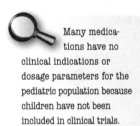 Many medications have no clinical indications or dosage parameters for the pediatric population because children have not been included in clinical trials.

responsibility of the healthcare professional ordering or administering medication to be aware of these dose parameters, which are readily available from package inserts or drug reference books, including the hospital formulary.

Pharmacokinetics

Concentration of drug at the desired site of action is affected by developmental **pharmacokinetics**, as well as intensity and duration of action. These are affected differently than in the adult population, with the greatest differences primarily in neonates and infants. After infancy, organ and system maturity reduce the pharmacokinetic risks. Serum drug levels remain elevated as a factor of delayed **elimination**, resulting in more intense and more prolonged response to medication. Increased sensitivity to medication in infants and neonates is related to

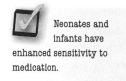

Neonates and infants have enhanced sensitivity to medication.

five immature physical processes: absorption, distribution (via circulation), blood-brain barrier, metabolism, and excretion.

Absorption

Drug **absorption** is affected by differences in gastric emptying times, which are irregular in the infant. Subcutaneous and intramuscular absorption is irregular in the neonate, as well. These very young children are at greater risk for toxicity from transdermally

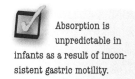

Absorption is unpredictable in infants as a result of inconsistent gastric motility.

or topically administered medication because of thin skin, high capillary distribution and differences in subcutaneous fat distribution, facilitating very rapid absorption.

Distribution

Drugs that commonly are highly bound with protein in the adult circulatory system, demonstrate significantly less protein binding in infants and neonates. Serum albumin levels are lower in infants than in adults, and endogenous compounds in the infant are more competitive for binding sites. So, infants experience relatively higher serum levels of unbound drug, resulting in greater risk for toxicity.

The immature **blood-brain barrier**, in infants and neonates, presents another risk in medication administration. This immature barrier results in greater access to the central nervous system (CNS), impacting CNS function.

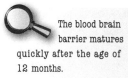

The blood brain barrier matures quickly after the age of 12 months.

Metabolism

Metabolic activity in the liver is slower in neonates, and to a lesser degree, in infants. This decrease in hepatic **metabolism** changes conversion of drugs in the liver to active or inactive metabolites. Slowed metabolism to active metabolites results in a decrease in drug activity, while slowed metabolism to inactive metabolites results in increased intensity and duration of action.

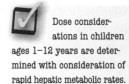

Dose considerations in children ages 1–12 years are determined with consideration of rapid hepatic metabolic rates.

Children over the age of one year through the age of 12 years usually metabolize medication more rapidly than adults.

Excretion

Renal function is reduced at birth, resulting in slowed excretion of medication, enhancing both duration and intensity of activity. This increases the risks of toxicity and accidental overdose.

Drug Choices

NSAIDs, acetaminophen, and salicylates like aspirin are appropriate for use in this client population, with adjustment for the correct dose. These are useful for mild to moderate pain and will also help with fever reduction. An NSAID or acetaminophen would be a more appropriate choice. This vital information should be shared with all parents of small children.

 Never use aspirin (salicylates) for children with viral symptoms, flu-like symptoms, or fever because of the risk of developing Reye's syndrome

In the case of more severe pain, or after procedures in which severe pain can be expected, opioids are a safe and effective medication choice to use in children. As with all clients receiving opioids, careful monitoring for side effects, excessive sedation, or respiratory depression is necessary. Positioning the very small or sedated child to maintain a patent airway is an important consideration. Treating for unpleasant side effects such as nausea and vomiting is also essential in this age group. As with adults, including an NSAID in the medication profile when possible can increase pain relief or prevention and may reduce the amount of opioid necessary.

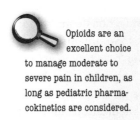

Opioids are an excellent choice to manage moderate to severe pain in children, as long as pediatric pharmacokinetics are considered.

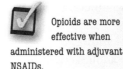

Opioids are more effective when administered with adjuvant NSAIDs.

Adjuvant medications to potential opioid use to promote relaxation, sedation, or reduce side effects are a third medication type to include in the plan of care. Local anesthetics, such as EMLA cream, are good choices to prevent procedure-related pain.

 An important goal in pain management for children is prevention, instead of relief for pain that has already occurred.

Choices for Administration

Routes of administration depend on a wide variety of factors in this population. Oral administration is appropriate when the child can safely swallow, when there is no need for rapid titration, and when oral intake is allowed. One other factor when choosing oral administration is the level of cooperation offered by the client. Children who resist oral medication and make it a continual battle to provide medication may require another administration route. It is important to remember that absorption of orally administered medications in neonates and infants may be erratic due to differences in gastric emptying time of pH.

Rectal administration is a very poor choice in neonates and infants as the result of incomplete sphincter control, the presence of feces in the rectum, and greater frequency of bowel movements than in older children or adults. Rectal absorption is commonly erratic and inconsistent in the very young. Toddlers may react negatively, perceiving this route as very invasive and confusing at a time when toilet training is in progress. Older age groups may also perceive it as invasive because of boundary, developmental, and sexuality issues.

Subcutaneous or intramuscular injections are also administration choices in children, but because they are also a cause of pain, they should be chosen only when absolutely necessary, especially with children younger than school age. Intramuscular injection in neonates results in a much slower absorption rate; however, intramuscular absorption is much faster in infants than in older children.

Intravenous (IV) administration is a good alternative when rapid titration of medication is necessary or when other routes are unacceptable. Use of a local anesthetic prior to intravenous insertion is desirable for this population. The IV site must be well protected in younger children, who do not understand its purpose and cannot be reasoned with or instructed not to tug at it. Peripheral intravenous lines are often difficult to achieve on neonates and infants because they have large amounts of subcutaneous fat in the arms and legs. One alternative is use of a superficial scalp vein, but this can be very distressing to parents.

Less invasive alternatives, such as administration across a mucous membrane, are becoming popular when caring for children. One excellent example is the fentanyl oralet (transmucosal fentanyl citrate), which is used to induce conscious sedation prior to procedures like closed reduction of a fracture. The opioid analgesic is supplied as a flavored lozenge and mounted on a handle like a lollipop. When the child sucks on the lozenge, the fentanyl citrate is absorbed through the mucosal tissues and gastrointestinal tract.

Patient-controlled analgesia (PCA) pumps are useful in older school-age children and adolescents. They are especially effective in these two groups by allowing the real sense of control over pain relief. They are also very useful for adolescents who are unwilling to verbalize pain needs. A PCA pump is not useful in younger children who cannot learn its use; it should not be considered acceptable for parents to administer IV medication as this would risk a narcotic overdose.

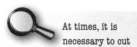 At times, it is necessary to cut a suppository in half to administer the required dose. Most suppositories should be split down the middle the long way, because medication is usually dispersed in the back of the tablet, with the head being glycerin or another inert material. Unfortunately, this leaves a long sliver that may be difficult to insert without breaking. A few extra minutes of refrigeration may make it easier to handle. Don't forget to share this information with parents, who may have to give their children suppositories at home.

CASE STUDY REVISITED

After verifying that Brian's last meal was more than 7 hours ago, conscious sedation is instituted using a fentanyl pop, administered buccally. As Brian relaxes, the orthopedist rapidly realigns the bone ends, and applies a splint. Although Brian cries out as the bones are manipulated, the nurse assures his father that Brian likely will not remember the procedure.

Brian appears very uncomfortable on awakening. Although the nurse intends to administer an opioid for pain relief, Brian's father is worried about giving Brian "serious drugs." The pediatric clinical nurse specialist (CNS) is called for a consultation. The CNS explains the safety and efficacy of using opioids in children. She administers one dose to Brian and helps his father place an ice pack over the splint. In her discussion with Brian's father and the staff nurse, the CNS explains that pain relief and hydration are two important goals for clients like Brian. Dehydration frequently exacerbates nausea and vomiting.

PHYSIOLOGICAL STRATEGIES FOR PAIN MANAGEMENT IN CHILDREN

Physiological strategies for this client population include the use of touch, massage, and physical contact; application of heat and cold; changes in position; and activity or exercise. Infants and toddlers crave contact with their mothers. Having Mom hold or snuggle the baby helps in providing comfort, security, and trust, and promotes reduction of tension. Gentle, rhythmic stroking and superficial massage is useful in all pediatric stages, but permission and explanations are necessary with older school-age children and adolescents, who have a strong sense of privacy about their bodies. Deep massage should only be used when there is no risk of bleeding or embolization.

BEHAVIORAL APPROACHES TO PAIN MANAGEMENT IN CHILDREN

Behavioral strategies in the pediatric client depend heavily on the developmental stage of the client. Neonates and infants are egocentric, with presence of a mother figure as a source of comfort. Allowing the infant to be held even during an invasive procedure increases the sense of comfort. A quiet environment and soft verbal stimulation such as singing or humming can provide distraction and soothe an anxious or crying infant. Toddlers also respond to this approach, but when they become overly active as a response to pain, holding them seems restrictive, resulting in further increases in activity. Although toddlers are beginning to verbalize, they can comprehend only the most basic instruction. Don't try to reason with a toddler. Give quiet verbal commands, and keep the environment quiet and nonthreatening.

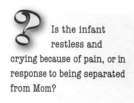
Is the infant restless and crying because of pain, or in response to being separated from Mom?

  Never try to reason with a toddler!

Invasive procedures for all age groups in the pediatric population should be done in a specific place, especially away from the bedside in an inpatient facility, to provide a safe place.

Preschool-age children are more responsive to words and actions that take into account their sense of magical thinking. Because this age group has fear of mutilation and is just beginning to establish body image boundaries, invasive procedures provoke anxiety. A well-placed bandage after any invasive procedure or injury, no matter how small, will prevent leaks, maintain body integrity, and provide a concrete notice of the event. Behavioral approaches with preschoolers should also be aimed very simply at helping the child to understand that he or she is not to blame for an illness or trauma.

School-age children and adolescents need to maintain a sense of control and privacy. Giving them *realistic* choices concerning treatment, timing, and perhaps route of administration may result in greater compliance with a plan of care. This age group should definitely be included in designing their own plan of care. They are capable of learning many of the behavioral approaches to pain management that are useful in the adult population. It is very important to remember that they are in the process of achieving very different and important developmental tasks and should not be treated like an adult. School-age children are excellent gatherers of information and are sensitive to truth-telling. It is important to be honest and retain their trust. They and adolescents have already begun to establish individual coping behaviors. They should be encouraged to use familiar coping strategies.

Family Considerations

Managing pain in the pediatric client is an interactive process involving healthcare professionals, parents, and children. When caring for the **family** as a unit, it is important to remember not to overwhelm a parent with tasks or responsibilities. For a parent, seeing his or her child in pain is a significantly stressful event. Trust and information provided by the healthcare professional will help to mediate some of that stress. Feelings

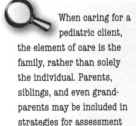 When caring for a pediatric client, the element of care is the family, rather than solely the individual. Parents, siblings, and even grandparents may be included in strategies for assessment and treatment.

of helplessness or failure make it worse. When identifying the plan of care, consider the parent along with the child. Set goals that are mutually agreeable and maintain a dialogue. Successful pain management occurs with successful interaction.

CASE STUDY RESOLVED

After a second dose of opioid in the emergency room, Brian began drinking water in amounts adequate for hydration. Before removing his IV though, the nurse wanted to be certain that oral pain medication will be adequate to relieve pain. Confident that his pain is well relieved, the nurse removes the IV and prepares Brian for discharge.

CHAPTER 9 • REVIEW QUESTIONS

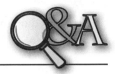

1. Which of the following is true regarding pain in children?
    A. Children have poorly developed nociceptors, so they do not frequently experience severe pain
    B. Pain management in children is similar to management in adults
    C. Pain management in children is frequently more challenging than in adults
    D. Children metabolize medications more quickly than adults

2. Which assessment parameter is essential in evaluating a pediatric client for pain management?
    A. Height and weight
    B. Developmental stage
    C. Social support
    D. All of the above

3. Behaviors used to express pain in children:
    A. Always involve regression in developmental stage
    B. Frequently seem unrelated to the source of pain
    C. Do not differ from behaviors seen in adults
    D. Are unreliable and should not be considered as part of pain assessment

4. Acute pain in children:
    A. Is always the result of trauma
    B. May be related to illness, intervention, or trauma
    C. Is less commonly seen than chronic pain
    D. Is seen only in specific healthcare settings

5. Use of medication administered on a PRN or as-needed basis for children with pain:
    A. Frequently results in poor pain management because of inappropriate assessment
    B. Is restricted to use only in critical care settings
    C. Provides excellent pain management
    D. Is never used as an alternative in planning that client's care

6. The first step in designing a plan for pain management in pediatric clients is:
   A. Height and weight
   B. Interview with parents, grandparents, and siblings
   C. Offering distraction and play therapy
   D. A complete and thorough assessment

7. Preschool-age children, although often able to verbalize their pain, frequently do not report it accurately as a result of all of the following except:
   A. Fear
   B. Magical thinking
   C. Concerns about bodily mutilation
   D. Lack of maternal trust

8. Safe and routine pediatric doses of medication are:
   A. Always half of the appropriate adult dose
   B. Specific to each medication
   C. Never shared with parents
   D. Found on the label of unit-dosed packages

9. Use of opioid medications with small children may result in sedation. The *most important* nursing intervention for these small clients is to:
   A. Position the child to maintain a patent airway
   B. Not use adjuvant medications to treat unpleasant side effects
   C. Caution against operating heavy machinery
   D. Reduce the dose of medication until sedation is no longer apparent

10. Rectal administration of medication is frequently most appropriate in which age group?
    A. Toddlers
    B. Adolescents
    C. Preschool-age children
    D. None of the above

ANSWERS AND RATIONALES

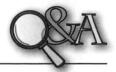

1. **C.** Pain management in children is frequently more challenging than in adults because of physical issues such as pharmacokinetics, as well as psychosocial and developmental considerations.

2. **D.** All should be considered.

3. **B.** Frequently seem unrelated to the source of pain, especially with diminished verbal skills or magical thinking.

4. **B.** Illness, intervention, or trauma may all result in acute episodes of pain in children; chronic pain is much less common.

5. **A.** Poor assessment leads to problems with administration of analgesics or opioids for pain management, especially when the medication is ordered on PRN. A PRN dosing schedule treats pain rather than attempts to keep the client relatively pain-free.

6. **D.** As with any pain management plan, a complete and thorough assessment is essential.

7. **D.** Fear, magical thinking, and concerns about bodily mutilation all interfere with pain assessment in the preschool-age child.

8. **B.** Doses are driven by pediatric pharmacokinetics and are specific to each medication.

9. **A.** Opioids may compromise a client's ability to maintain an airway.

10. **D.** Rectal administration is not considered efficient or reliable in any of these age groups.

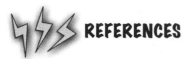 **REFERENCES**

Acute Pain Management Guideline Panel. (1992). *Acute pain management in infants, children, and adolescents: operative procedures. Quick reference guide for clinicians. No. 1a. AHCPR Pub No. 92-0019.* Rockville, MD: Agency for Health Care Policy and Research, Public Health Service, U.S. Department of Health and Human Services.

Acute Pain Management Guideline Panel. (1992). *Acute pain management: operative or medical procedures and trauma. AHCPR Pub No. 92-0032.* Rockville, MD: Agency for Health Care Policy and Research, Public Health Service, U.S. Department of Health and Human Services.

Finely, G. A., McGrath, P., & Chambers, C. T. (2006). *Bringing pain relief to children: treatment approaches.* Totowa, NJ: Humana Press.

Karch, A. M. (2006). *2007 Lippincott's nursing drug guide.* Philadelphia: Lippincott Williams & Wilkins.

McCaffery, M., & Pasero, C. (1999). *Pain: clinical manual.* St. Louis, MO: Mosby.

Schechter, N. L., Berde, B. L., & Yaster, M. (2003). *Pain in infants, children and adolescents.* Philadelphia: Lippincott Williams & Wilkins.

Wong, D. L. (2007). *Wong's nursing care of infants and children* (8th ed.). St. Louis, MO: Mosby.

Wong, D. L., & Perry, S. E. (2006). *Maternal child nursing care* (3rd ed.). St. Louis, MO: Mosby.

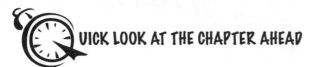

The growth of the elderly as a segment of the national population challenges healthcare providers to respond to their specific issues. Factors encouraging the growth of the elderly population include the graying of the baby boomers, extension of the life span, improvements in screening for and treatment of disease, and economic shifts. Some specific needs of this population stem from their higher predisposition to illness, both chronic and acute, as well as higher rates of terminal illnesses. Related to their increased healthcare needs is the problem of pain in the elderly population, which is a frequent occurrence with multiple chronic as well as acute conditions.

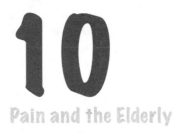

10

Pain and the Elderly

TERMS
- [ ] age-related changes
- [ ] biotransformation
- [ ] confusion
- [ ] dementia
- [ ] depression
- [ ] elderly
- [ ] immobility
- [ ] sedation

CASE STUDY

Mrs. R., a 78-year-old woman, has lived in an assisted living facility since her husband died 3 years ago. Her children live in other states and are not actively involved in her care. Although Mrs. R. suffers from early-stage Alzheimer's disease, she is very active in the community and is able to manage her own activities of daily living with minimal supervision. She has been complaining to the nurses of right-sided abdominal pain and flank pain for 2 days. They have observed her rubbing or holding her right side as well. On assessment, she is febrile, diaphoretic, and reports having several bouts of diarrhea over the past 36 hours. Her appetite is very poor, and she appears dehydrated. Upon examination, her lower right quadrant is tender to touch. She is positive for guarding and abdominal rigidity. Bowel sounds are diminished throughout.

 ## AGING AND THE EXPERIENCE OF PAIN

There is no reason to believe that the elderly client does not experience pain, or that the pain experience is reduced with aging. No normal physiological changes associated with aging are responsible for diminishing pain sensations. The **elderly** do experience changes in the natural aging process that put them at higher risk for injury and illness with related pain, as well as changes that may interfere with attempts at interventions for pain relief. By specifically targeting assessment and intervention techniques to the individual elderly client in pain, successful pain relief is a possibility.

 Multiple physical changes occur with aging. They may be a part of the natural aging process or may be related to illness or trauma. It is important to consider these changes when planning interventions.

 Never assume all elderly individuals are the same.

Assessing the Elderly Client for Pain

Assessment is vitally important to attempt to identify the source and type of pain, especially with the complication of multiple problems that the elderly client may experience. **Confusion** or **dementia**, hearing or vision loss, or isolation may further confuse assessment attempts. Changes in mental status commonly associated with aging, including senescence or Alzheimer's disease, complicate manifestation of acute and chronic pain. The client may not vocalize pain or may act in ways frequently associated with pain. Alternate and client-specific assessment strategies must be used for these clients to determine the presence of pain and the success of interventions.

 Normal and illness-related physiological changes exist in the elderly client who is experiencing pain. These changes must be considered in assessment and intervention strategies, especially when using pharmacological interventions.

 It is essential that the mental status of the elderly client be considered in the assessment process, as it may interfere with adequate pain management.

Causes of Pain in the Elderly

Age-related Changes

What causes pain in the elderly client? The causes are as varied as the clients themselves. Pain may be an acute phenomenon associated with trauma, injury, illness, or surgery. **Age-related changes** in visual acuity, hearing, mobility, balance, and judgment increase the elderly client's propensity for accidents and traumatic injury.

Loss in body mass—muscular, fatty, or subcutaneous tissue—results in the potential for more severe injury than for younger clients in the same traumatic instance. Osteoporosis, a loss of bone density, results in the potential for fractures. Subcutaneous tissue loss often results in fine, tissue-paper-thin skin that is easily torn. Even slight dehydration causes changes in skin turgor, which can result in easier or more extensive injury.

Despite weight gain in older clients, subcutaneous tissue and muscle mass are lost, increasing risk of injury.

Injuries to the skin, subcutaneous tissues, muscles, tendons, ligaments, or bones may result in an inflammatory response, mediated by the immune system. Breaks in the skin or mucous membranes are potential avenues for the development of infection. Infections also result in immune and inflammatory responses. Chemical mediators of the inflammatory response are also chemical mediators in the pain process, so elderly clients at risk for these problems are at increased risk for pain. Normal changes in the aging process *do not* involve a breakdown or weakening of the immune system, so inflammation continues to be a natural response to injury in the elderly client.

 Age-related changes increase potential for injury occurrence and severity.

Vascular Changes

Manifestation of pain may occur or change with vascular changes associated with aging. Anginal pain or intermittent claudication may accompany arterial insufficiency related to atherosclerosis or hypertension. Peripheral neuropathies may reduce or completely inhibit the sensation of pain in the affected extremities, thus restricting the protective mechanisms associated with pain. Neuropathies are frequently associated with venous changes, diabetes mellitus, or use of certain neurotoxic medications. Peripheral neuropathies are generally not reversible. Pain sensation may be masked by the use of prescribed or over-the-counter medication. Many elderly clients use pain medication for chronic conditions such as osteoarthritis. Even the use of aspirin as a cardioprotective may reduce the pain response. For this reason, it is very important to document a comprehensive medication history when assessing an elderly client for pain.

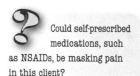 Could self-prescribed medications, such as NSAIDs, be masking pain in this client?

Acute or Chronic Medical Conditions

Multiple medical conditions that occur more commonly as the client ages are related to increased incidences of pain. Chronic conditions, including osteoarthritis, result in pain that may significantly affect the elderly client's quality of life and is responsible for self-medication as well as increased visits to the doctor or nurse practitioner. Cancers are more common in the elderly client as well. With improvements in treatment and detec-

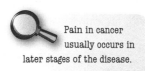 Pain in cancer usually occurs in later stages of the disease.

tion of many types of cancer, the associated pain is often in the chronic phase of the illness. Pre-existing or chronic illnesses may mask manifestations of acute pain or delay appropriate intervention for acute pain.

Healthcare-related Causes of Pain

Frequent interface with the healthcare professional is yet another reason for the experience of pain for the elderly client. Painful diagnostic procedures, surgical procedures, treatments, and rehabilitation all account for instances of iatrogenic pain. Prior to certain invasive procedures, medications used for the treatment of chronic pain that interfere with blood clotting, such as NSAIDs or aspirin, must be curtailed. It is important to be proactive in identifying alternate pain relief interventions appropriate for the client to use in the absence of his or her usual relief measures.

 ## PHARMACOKINETIC CONSIDERATIONS

Normal and illness-related physiological changes in the elderly client experiencing pain must be considered in determining intervention strategies, especially when using pharmacological interventions.

Absorption

Oral Administration

Routes of administration should be carefully considered in relation to age-related changes. Oral routes can be affected by changes in swallowing ability, changes in the amount of oral secretions, and changes in digestion. Carefully assess the client's ability to swallow tablets. If swallowing is a problem, consider breaking the tablet into smaller pieces or crushing it to administer it with thickened liquids such as applesauce or dissolved in water or juice. Tablets that are designed for timed release or with enteric coatings should not be broken or crushed. Many medications are available in liquid or suspension forms as an alternative to tablets.

 Enteric coated or time-release tablets should never be crushed or broken.

To assist the client in swallowing tablets, have him or her sit upright if possible. Place the tablet at the front of the tongue for better control.

If the tablet is placed at the back of the mouth, it is sometimes more difficult to swallow. Swallowing is easier with only one tablet at a time. Clients who take multiple medications at one time often attempt to swallow them all at once. This practice could result in aspiration or choking for the client who has difficulty swallowing. After administering pills to an elderly client, examine the mouth to assure they have been swallowed. This could prevent choking later, in addition to making certain that the medicine will not be found on the floor or in the bedding later.

 Placing pills at the very back of the mouth increases the risk of aspiration.

Clients who are dehydrated or complain of a dry mouth (such as elderly clients on antihypertensive medications or diuretics) may complain of difficulty swallowing pills because they "stick" to the oral mucosa. Giving the client a small sip of juice or water prior to giving the pills frequently helps with this complaint. Clients with hiatal hernias or acid reflux often complain that pills cause an increase in discomfort. Reduced stomach motility may interfere with timely absorption of medication taken orally.

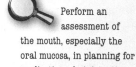 Perform an assessment of the mouth, especially the oral mucosa, in planning for medication administration for the elderly client.

Sublingual or Transbuccal Administration

Sublingual (medication placed under the tongue) or transbuccal administration—medication absorbed across the buccal membrane (mucous membranes under the tongue or between the gums and cheek)—can be problematic because of dry mouth, fragile membranes, dentures, or poor circulation. Clients with a dry mouth, which may occur as a natural change in aging or from medications or medical conditions, may experience difficulty with medications administered via this route. Insufficient moisture may slow or prevent the tablet from dissolving. The tablets may become stuck or may damage already fragile mucous membranes. Damage to the oral mucous membranes will result in pain and inflammation. Inflammation will interfere with transbuccal absorption.

Dental appliances may get in the way of tablet placement. Tablets may also become caught under dentures, causing injury. Some medications are now available as sprays for transbuccal administration. Finally, in the elderly client with swallowing difficulties and/or mentation changes, placement of pills under the tongue or between the gum and cheek may present an aspiration hazard.

Medications available in spray form may be difficult for the older adult to manage if manual dexterity is reduced by arthritic changes or neuropathies.

Transcutaneous Administration

Transcutaneous or transdermal absorption of medication may be affected by more rapid metabolism, thinning of skin or subcutaneous tissue, or poor circulation. Many pain management medications are prescribed for elderly adults using this route, including nitropaste and fentanyl. Clients who are febrile will absorb and metabolize medication across the skin more quickly. This results in poor pain relief prior to the next administration. Loss of subcutaneous tissue or poor peripheral circulation causes poor absorption and movement of the medication into circulation.

When placing transdermal medication on elderly clients, choose a spot on the trunk, avoiding the limbs. Monitor the client for fever. Assess the area of placement for pallor or mottling, signs of poor circulation. Avoid scarred areas or open areas, such as skin tears or abrasions.

Patches that use adhesives or tape to hold the patches in place should be used and removed with caution, as elderly clients' skin may be fragile and easily torn.

Subcutaneous Administration

Subcutaneous injection is an option with similar drawbacks for use in the elderly population. Loss of subcutaneous tissue reduces areas for the medication to deposit. Changes in peripheral circulation may reduce transport of the medication into systemic circulation, reducing effective pain control. Careful assessment of the injection site for symptoms of circulatory compromise, including atrophy, pallor, and mottling, will reduce some of the transport problems. Choosing a site for injection on the trunk, especially the abdomen (avoiding the umbilicus or any areas of varicosity), is also beneficial to improve pain control.

Some specific advantages to using subcutaneous injection include the fact that the needle is small and fine, making a relatively painless injection technique. Bruising or bleeding are infrequent complications. This form of administration is a technique that can readily be taught to clients and their families.

Intramuscular Administration

Intramuscular injection is problematic in the elderly client who has lost muscle tissue to atrophy, wasting, or loss of body mass. Careful choice of site should consider the volume of medication to be injected, as decreased muscle mass reduces the area for storage or deposit of medication. Atrophy caused by circulatory insufficiencies is a good indicator that transport of the injected medication to central circulation will be poor. Finally, intramuscular injections may be extremely painful, especially when administered to a muscle that is not in a state of relaxation. Proper positioning and relaxation techniques are good aids to preventing muscle tension.

Rectal Administration

Rectal administration is often a reasonable choice when the oral route is not a possibility for reasons such as nausea and vomiting or difficulty swallowing. Some particular considerations when using this route for the elderly client include comfort, safety, bowel habits, and cardiac history. Suppositories are made up of inert solid material that melts, such as glycerin, allowing the medication to be absorbed across the rectal mucosa. The suppository must be retained in the rectal vault long enough for melting and absorption. Clients suffering from diarrhea or rectal irritation may not be able to resist the urge to defecate, thus expelling the suppository before the medication is absorbed. Clients with hemorrhoids often complain of intense discomfort when suppositories are inserted. Elderly clients may have difficulty lying in a position to facilitate insertion. Using the rectal route for self-administration of pain medication is repellent to some clients. Peripheral neuropathies or osteoarthritis diminish manual dexterity, making handling the suppository and insertion difficult. Stimulation of the vasovagal response when medication is inserted rectally is potentially dangerous to clients with a cardiac history. Even absent of a history of cardiac problems, vagal stimulation may result in a drop in cardiac rate and blood pressure, resulting in syncope.

Assess the elderly client carefully before using this route, and provide safety measures, including protection from falls and other consequences of syncope, as well as ready access to a bathroom, commode, or bedpan should the rectal insertion stimulate a strong urge for a bowel movement. It is important to know that colostomy stomas can be used for insertion of rectal medication. Absorption across the mucous membranes of ileostomy or urinary diversion stomas is less certain, primarily because of the consistent nature of the drainage.

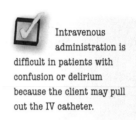

How can dignity and safety be maintained for the older adult being medicated using the rectal route?

Intravenous Administration

Intravenous (IV) access allows for medication to be administered directly into the circulatory system. It allows for rapid pain relief, but the medication is not stored, resulting in relief of a shorter duration. IV access in elderly clients can be difficult because of poor peripheral circulation, dehydration, or noncompliance. A central line is a possibility in these cases but is more difficult to care for (especially out of the acute care environment), has the potential for complications such as hemorrhage or infection, and is more difficult and painful to insert.

Intravenous administration is difficult in patients with confusion or delirium because the client may pull out the IV catheter.

Metabolism

Biotransformation

In addition to physical changes that affect the choice of routes of administration, changes that affect the metabolism or storage of medication within the body occur as a part of aging. Age-related changes in the liver could affect the **biotransformation** of certain medications. Biotransformation refers to the conversion of medications to chemical states, which are more bioavailable for use within the body. Transformation time increases, resulting in longer elevated serum levels of drugs. Dosage intervals should be increased and maximum doses should be carefully adhered to, preventing damage to the liver from accumulation of drugs or drug metabolites. Acetaminophen is one excellent example of a drug that is widely used by this population for pain control and is transformed in the liver.

Despite the fact that acetaminophen is readily available at low cost over-the-counter, it is frequently a poor choice for self-medication in elders.

Excretion

Age-related changes within the kidneys affect renal clearance and excretion of drugs and drug metabolites, also resulting in longer periods of optimal or elevated serum drug levels. These changes may be obvious as signs and symptoms of mild, moderate, or severe renal failure, or they can be occult. Dehydration exacerbates this phenomenon. Decreasing the dose and increasing dose intervals will accommodate this change. It is very important to assess the client frequently, not only for adequate pain relief but also for signs and symptoms related to expected side effects and toxicity. Morphine sulfate is a good example of a frequently used medication for pain that is cleared through the kidneys.

 # OTHER CHANGES COMMON IN AGING

Immune Function and Pain Management

Normal or expected physiological changes in the elderly client do not include an expected decrease in immunity; however, this is a problem experienced by many elderly clients. A decrease in effective function of the immune system can be related to many factors. Malnutrition or a decrease in intake of food and fluids as well as various disease processes has been implicated in immunocompromise. Use of medications as treatment for various comorbidities may cause a reduction in function of the elderly client's immune response. Some of these medications include antineoplastics, cardiac medications, steroids, other hormone replacements, and the use of antibiotics. Reduced immune response should be evaluated and considered when selecting interventions for pain as well as administration alternatives. Use of narcotics or other interventions that may reduce mobility in the immunocompromised client carry the potential for complications of immobility such as pneumonia or skin breakdown.

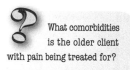

What comorbidities is the older client with pain being treated for?

Changes in Mobility

The elderly client frequently exhibits alterations in mobility. **Immobility** or other potential complications can be exacerbated or related to medications used for pain relief, or even to nonpharmacological interventions for pain. These complications include skin breakdown, constipation, urinary tract infection, deep vein thrombosis (DVT) and embolization, pneumonia, problems with digestion and respiration, isolation, and depression. Use of sedating medication such as opioids may decrease a client's already compromised mobility. Opioids can cause or exacerbate constipation and nausea. They may depress respiration. Use of NSAIDs can cause bleeding dyscrasias or be difficult to use with anticoagulants for treating DVTs. Changes in mobility may reduce positioning or activity options as nonpharmacological interventions.

 Appropriate pain management may prevent or reduce immobility and its potential multiple complications.

Mobility and Complications of Pain Management

By assessing the client's mobility and potential for problems initially and throughout the period that pain relief interventions are used, complications can be prevented or treated and resolved at early stages. One example is bowel status. Assessment of the client's baseline or premorbid bowel habits provides target criteria for comfort while using opioids. Increasing dietary fiber and fluid intake, and using a bulk laxative and stool softener as a bowel regimen will prevent constipation and impaction as complications of immobility and medication side effects. Continued assessment for the efficacy of both pain relief and bowel regiment with changes in the plan of care as appropriate are necessary throughout the intervention period.

 Always consider prevention of constipation as part of an opioid treatment protocol.

Changes in mentation, including confusion, anxiety, and depression, occur in the elderly, complicating both assessment for discomfort as well as alternatives for pain management. These changes will be addressed later in this chapter.

CASE STUDY REVISITED

After further testing, a diagnosis of small bowel obstruction is made, and Mrs. R. is admitted to the hospital for surgical intervention. Postoperatively, Mrs. R. remains pain-free with around-the-clock doses of intramuscular morphine sulfate. Although use of a PCA pump was considered, the emergency nature of her surgery and her diagnosis of Alzheimer's disease were contraindications. PRN dosing of narcotics postoperatively would have aimed at relieving pain, rather than preventing it.

MEDICATION STRATEGIES IN PAIN MANAGEMENT FOR ELDERLY CLIENTS

Choosing and administering medications as interventions for pain in the elderly client is complicated by many of the physiological changes that accompany aging or the comorbidities frequently seen in this population. A wide variety of medication classes are available for use in these clients with minimal restrictions.

Acute Pain Management

When managing acute pain, it is important to attempt to identify the source or cause of the pain and treat it, if possible. Acute pain may occur in the elderly population more frequently in addition to chronic pain syndromes. Each type of pain should be considered carefully so that appropriate treatment can be used. Medications used for one type or source of pain may not be effective for another source or type.

When planning for administration of appropriate medications, the step approach described by the clinical practice guidelines should be used. NSAIDs or salicylates are good alternatives for mild to moderate pain, with the *addition* of opioids as an alternative for more severe or unrelieved pain. Disease-specific medications for pain management should also be included in the plan of care. However, a complete medication-use history is essential when planning for pharmacological intervention for pain in the elderly client. Multiple comorbidities may exist, and the elderly client may take multiple medications, enhancing the potential for medication interactions.

 A complete medication use history is critical in planning a pain management strategy.

Self-prescribed Medications

When taking a medication history, remember to include medications prescribed by a physician or nurse practitioner as well as self-medication. These self-prescribed medications may include symptom management with over-the-counter preparations for pain, constipation, heartburn, or a multitude of other symptoms. It may also include prescription medications that do not belong to this client. Recreational drugs should also be included in this profile. It is an unwise assumption that because the client is "old," he or she is exempt from using recreational or illicit drugs.

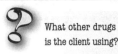 What other drugs is the client using?

Complications of Drug Interactions

All drugs and medications used can contribute to the problem of medication interactions. Some complications seen in the elderly population when medication interactions occur include respiratory distress, dizziness, syncope, fatigue, sedation, constipation, dehydration, changes in blood pressure or cardiac output, changes in serum drug levels, and cardiac symptoms. Medication interactions can be mildly problematic or life-threatening. The elderly population has the most potential risk for medication interactions.

Side Effects

Care should also be taken when choosing a medication regimen for pain relief to avoid use of medications that may complicate or mimic some of the age-related changes. Previously, the effect of medications on mobility has been discussed. Many elderly clients who use narcotics, especially morphine, as a choice for pain management express dissatisfaction with sedation, drowsiness, and depression.

 Changes in pharmacokinetics in the older adult put them at greater risk for side effects.

Depression

Depression is not a side effect of opioids, but it can be a significant symptom of pain, especially chronic pain. If the client suffers from symptoms of depression, strategies to treat the depression should be part of the plan of care.

Sedation

Clients who doze or nap when alone in a quiet room but are easily awakened and engaged by company or activity are not overly sedated by their pain medication. Frequently, clients who have suffered sleep deprivation because of their pain, illness, or hospitalization will sleep for long periods once their pain has been relieved. This is not medication-induced **sedation.** Generally, in this case, the prolonged periods of sleeping will be reduced in 24 to 48 hours.

If sedation is unacceptable to the client, attempt to decrease the dose of medication and/or increase the dosage interval. Carefully assess for pain relief while manipulating the dose of medication. If a change in type or classification of medication is necessary to alleviate sedation or other side effects, use an equianalgesic table or formula to ensure adequate medication.

 It is not appropriate to withhold opioid medication to reduce sedation when family members visit.

Managing Side Effects

Side effects that occur from medications that are providing adequate pain relief can be treated independently, rather than changing an already effective medication. Some side effects about which the elderly frequently complain, in addition to sedation, are light-headedness or dizziness, gastrointestinal problems, and itching. Clients using opioids, anesthetic agents, cardiac medications, and neuroleptics may report feelings of light-headedness or a drop in blood pressure. Carefully assess the client for adequate hydration, as these symptoms can be related to or made worse by even moderate dehydration. Client teaching regarding safety is important when experiencing these symptoms.

 Safety is an important consideration when planning pain management strategies.

When using NSAIDs or aspirin, clients may report heartburn, abdominal pain, or reflux. Counsel the client not to take these medications on an empty stomach, as this increases the symptoms. Use of an antacid may be of some help. Assess that overdose is not a problem. Some medications are available with an enteric coating to protect the stomach (remember, these cannot be crushed or broken for administration). Be alert for signs and symptoms of gastric ulcers or gastrointestinal bleeding. Clients using these classes of medication may also complain of nausea, which may be relieved by a bland diet and by not taking the medications when the stomach is empty. Nausea and sometimes vomiting is more frequently associated with the use of narcotics, especially morphine. This can be managed with the use of a variety of antiemetics. Nausea is frequently a problem with these medications when oral intake is poor, especially when the medications are being administered orally. Codeine is a particular culprit in causing nausea. If antiemetic therapy is not appropriate or unsuccessful, then a change in medication or medication class should be considered. Constipation is another side effect associated with opioid use, which can be a problem for the elderly client. This has been discussed earlier in this chapter.

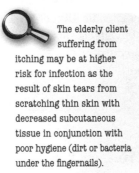 The elderly client suffering from itching may be at higher risk for infection as the result of skin tears from scratching thin skin with decreased subcutaneous tissue in conjunction with poor hygiene (dirt or bacteria under the fingernails).

Itching, with or without an accompanying rash, is another frequent complaint from elderly clients on many different types of pain medication. Although itching can sometimes be the first symptom in an anaphylactic response, usually accompanied by hives, it is normally an uncomfortable but not unsafe side effect. It can be managed with use of an antihistamine topically or systematically.

Side Effects and Age-related Changes

Elderly clients more frequently experience side effects from pain-relief medications. This is often a consequence of age-related changes, specifically renal or hepatic changes. Reducing the dose or increasing the dosage interval may offer relief from the side effects while maintaining adequate pain control. Client teaching regarding side effects and their management are essential in helping our elderly clients comply with the pain medication regimen.

NONPHARMACOLOGICAL OPTIONS FOR PAIN CONTROL IN ELDERS

Choosing methods of pain relief in addition to (adjunct) or instead of medication has become more and more popular in recent times. When identifying alternative interventions for pain, safety, acceptability to the client, and potential for a positive outcome must be considered. Practicing holistic, client-centered care and a move away from the medical model are stimuli to explore alternatives in pain management. A wide variety is available, which may be received with varied degrees of enthusiasm from the elderly client.

This client population has been treated for many years utilizing the medical model. They have experienced or been aware of multiple advances in medicine and healthcare science. If the client does not believe that an intervention will be successful, the chances of success are seriously diminished. With this in mind, presentation of nonpharmacological methods must be positive and professional. Establishment of a therapeutic presence or therapeutic relationship is valuable in utilizing nonpharmacological methods and may be a potent intervention for relief of pain as well. The therapeutic relationship helps in relieving anxiety, muscle tension, and stress. It assists the client to a more receptive state, making client teaching, relaxation, and guided imagery easier.

Massage, Heat and Cold Therapies

Cutaneous stimulation and the use of heat and cold are alternatives for pain relief that are familiar and successful to many elderly clients. Cutaneous stimulation includes light or deep massage. Massage can be at the site of pain or in another area of the body. Massage becomes a dangerous alternative if potential damage can be done, as when embolization is a threat.

Use of heat or cold may work by utilizing the gate control theory or may be useful in reducing inflammation, thereby reducing pain. Use of heat in areas of vascular insufficiency is contraindicated. Another particular danger when using heat as pain management in this population is the risk of burns. The elderly client may be unaware of extreme temperature because of peripheral neuropathies. Skin is more fragile, frequently with diminished protective subcutaneous fat. Hot compresses should be tested by another individual for appropriate temperature, and the elderly client should avoid unsupervised use of electronic heating pads.

As the result of age-related changes in skin and subcutaneous tissue, the older adult is at much greater risk for injury from applications of heat or cold.

Psychobehavioral Interventions

Distraction, relaxation, and positive use of leisure time are all realistic options, especially in adjunct pain management. Providing the elderly client with control over pain management will also enhance results. Self-scheduling administration of pain medications or use of a PCA pump are appropriate choices for the client who is not suffering from confusion or other altered mental states. Positioning and increased activity to reduce complications of immobility and frequent periods of rest is also useful. Client teaching to provide information about the causes of the pain as well as methods for pain relief is important to the elder, affording the potential for even greater control.

Finally, consider ethnic or cultural diversity in the expression and meaning of pain, as well as relief alternatives that are specific to the culture of the client. The elderly client may be particularly invested in historical or cultural alternatives. Nonpharmacological methods for pain control that are unacceptable or unbelievable to the client will be of little value. For this reason, client education is essential in successful choice and use of pain control other than or in addition to medication. These choices frequently are more successful in addition to rather than instead of pharmacological pain control.

PAIN MANAGEMENT FOR THE ELDERLY CLIENT WITH ALTERED MENTAL STATUS

Depression and confusion are two changes in mental status that may be seen in the elderly client. Neither of these are normal, age-related changes to be expected as part of the aging process. Identifying causes or exacerbating factors and treating the client for depression or confusion should be attempted. However, both confusion and depression may alter the ways in which a client expresses or experiences pain, as well as the efficacy of pain-relief interventions.

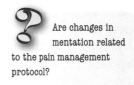 Are changes in mentation related to the pain management protocol?

Assessment criteria for pain in the client with mental status changes differ from those for other clients. Verbal expression of pain or requests for relief may not be evident. The client may not behave as one would expect a client in pain to behave. The depressed client may become even more withdrawn, with a flattened or angry affect. The confused client may exhibit either agitated or withdrawn behavior. Periods of confusion may get longer or the client may appear more confused than his or her baseline assessment. Physical indicators of increased pain may be the only clues. Increases in pulse, respiration, blood pressure; positional changes; guarding; or rigidity of the area of pain, pallor, and diaphoresis are all indicators of pain. Changes in behavior should be considered as indicators of pain. A medication review may indicate potential causes or enhancers of the behavioral changes. Use these cues when deciding to administer pain medication or other interventions, as well as assessing for the effectiveness of interventions provided. Signs and symptoms of pain in the client may be paradoxical and not what you would expect at all. Individualized plans of care for each client include specific assessment criteria and interventions for that particular client.

Depression

Depression may be an organic process, or it can be situational. Many clients may experience depression as the result of the diagnosis of an acute or chronic illness, or living with a chronic condition. Depression may also be related to isolation, reduced activity, immobility, or diminished ability for self-care. The client who is depressed appears saddened or presents a flat affect. Changes in eating and sleep patterns occur. Fatigue, loss of energy, and a diminished capacity for enjoyment, peace, or comfort are symptoms as well. The depressed client may not manifest symptoms or complaints about pain as readily. Pain may become quite severe before relief is sought out. For this reason, the client who is depressed should be engaged and assessed repeatedly for pain and the effectiveness of efforts aimed at pain relief. Depression does not cause physical pain, but pain can result in feelings of depression. Chronic pain often has depression as a complicating factor.

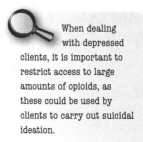

When dealing with depressed clients, it is important to restrict access to large amounts of opioids, as these could be used by clients to carry out suicidal ideation.

Confusion

Confusion is another mental status change seen in the elderly client. It can be related to a wide variety of client issues. Confusion may have an organic cause, such as Alzheimer's disease or organic brain syndrome. It may result from chronic or acute episodes of hypoxia, sleep deprivation, or be a side effect of medication such as morphine or general anesthesia. Elderly clients are more apt to become confused when removed from a familiar environment or routine. Careful assessment of the client's baseline mental status is important to facilitate removing factors that may cause or exacerbate confusion or forgetfulness. Confusion is commonly assessed initially by orientation to person, place, and time. When disoriented in one or more of these fields, the client may not remember how to seek out relief for pain, what the cause of pain might be, or who has helped with pain-relief interventions.

 ## CUES FOR COMPLIANCE

Interventions for pain relief or a plan of care that include medications as well as nonpharmacological approaches are only useful if the client is compliant with the proposed interventions. Medications that are unavailable, difficult to use, or have intolerable side effects cannot relieve pain when the client opts not to use them. Adjuvant approaches must be believable, available, and easy to use. When designing a pain management program include availability, believability, control, ease of use, and complete and available information.

When considering availability for the elderly client, the healthcare setting must be considered. In an institutional setting such as hospital or nursing home, the client should understand how to access an intervention through healthcare personnel. Many elderly clients resist calling the nurse for pain medication, instead waiting until the nurse makes rounds to avoid "bothering" him or her when busy. In this instance, more frequent trips to the bedside or offers for intervention should be a part of the plan of care. Outside of institutional settings, availability includes issues such as affordability of the intervention, where it can be purchased, who will transport it to the client, where it can be safely stored, the client's or family members' ability to administer it safely, and even who can open that child-proof cap!

 Never assume that medication is readily available.

When designing interventions for pain management, it is important that the client believe that the interventions will help relieve pain. Goals must be realistic. In some instances, complete pain relief is not a realistic option. Communication and understanding of this will help to prevent the client's impression of an intervention as a complete failure. Previous use of medications should be assessed, identifying pain medications that, when used previously, were unsuccess-

 Chances are, if an elderly client has previous experience with a pain management technique that failed, or even information from a relative or friend that a technique didn't work, that technique will be neither believable nor effective for that client.

ful or problematic. Potential side effects should be planned for from the outset of therapy. Be a cheerleader; help to convince the client that the interventions suggested will be helpful. Continual assessment will identify those interventions that do work. Listen closely to the client's doubts and fears.

Clients who have control over interventions for pain frequently have greater success with pain management. Build control and realistic choices for the client into the plan of care. Self-management of medication, timing, treatment schedules, when and how adjuvant therapies will be used, and who will provide assistance when necessary are all part of the plan. Consider mental status changes when building in appropriate and safe control for the client. Frequent mental status assessment is essential in the elderly client because of increased propensity toward medication-related confusion or sedation. A plan of care is continually evaluated and can be changed frequently as indicated by efficacy.

Interventions that are difficult to accomplish are frequently left unused. The client in pain has diminished energy and resources, and is easily exhausted. This principle is closely related to the discussion of availability above.

Finally, information concerning the interventions planned must be complete and available to the client, significant others, and the whole healthcare team. Misunderstanding of incomplete information can be the cause of failure in pain management. Think carefully about documentation techniques and assessment criteria. Verbal, written, and other forms of information are important for the client and significant others, especially as a reference when the nurse is not currently available. Considering details that will increase client compliance will increase the potential for successful pain management.

CASE STUDY RESOLVED

Within 3 days of surgery, Mrs. R. develops bowel sounds in all four quadrants, reports flatus, and is tolerating a regular diet. At this point, her opioid is changed to Percocet (acetaminophen and oxycodone) every 6 hours around-the-clock. In addition, she is prescribed a fiber laxative and encouraged to increase fluid intake. The nurse monitors her bowel status, and Mrs. R. continues to be pain-free.

CHAPTER 10 · REVIEW QUESTIONS

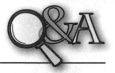

1. Pain in the elderly population is:
    A. A less frequent problem due to diminished sensation
    B. More common due to increased healthcare needs
    C. Difficult to manage due to widespread chronic malnutrition
    D. Successfully managed only by gerontology specialists

2. Considerations in choosing a route of administration for medication in the elderly include:
    A. Loss of subcutaneous tissue and muscle mass
    B. Noncompliance
    C. Hearing difficulties
    D. None of the above

3. Manifestations of pain related to vascular changes in the elderly include:
    A. Macular degeneration
    B. Osteoarthritic pain
    C. Intermittent claudication
    D. Pain related to ill-fitting dentures

4. Acute pain in the elderly client:
    A. Is always easily assessed
    B. May be masked by over-the-counter medication use
    C. Is responsive to NSAID therapy
    D. Rarely reflects the severity of illness or trauma

5. Changes in mental status associated with senility, dementia, or Alzheimer's disease may result in inadequate pain management because of:
    A. Masking of manifestations of acute pain
    B. Inability to perceive pain due to central nervous system changes
    C. Inability to vocalize or describe pain
    D. All of the above

6. Narcotic use in the elderly client should be carefully monitored because of which expected changes in physiology related to aging?
   A. Inability to swallow
   B. Changes in renal function, resulting in faster renal clearance
   C. Changes in liver function, resulting in longer elevated serum drug levels
   D. Restricted mobility, slowing drug metabolism

7. Including analgesic medication in the polypharmacy approach to medication in the elderly includes:
   A. Careful evaluation of all medications currently in use before adding analgesics
   B. Cautioning the elderly client to take different medications at specified time intervals
   C. Use of multiple pharmacies to fill existing prescriptions
   D. Relying on the elderly client to coordinate communication among all healthcare providers prescribing his or her medications

8. Elderly clients may describe heartburn or symptoms of reflux when using NSAIDs or aspirin therapy. The best intervention to suggest managing this symptom is:
   A. Take all medications with an 8-ounce glass of milk
   B. Cut tablets in half for easy swallowing
   C. Use enteric coated tablets, if they are available
   D. Restrict use of aspirin or NSAIDs until symptoms disappear

9. Use of heat as a nonpharmacological method of pain management should be monitored carefully because:
   A. An elderly person could easily be electrocuted using a heating pad
   B. An elderly person may be more susceptible to burns because of thin, frail skin and decreased subcutaneous tissue
   C. An elderly client is too confused to remember to use heat
   D. Heat is always the treatment of choice for pain related to vascular insufficiency

10. Which of the following are important to assess with long-term medication intervention for chronic pain?
    A. Mentation
    B. Nutrition
    C. Compliance
    D. All of the above

ANSWERS AND RATIONALES

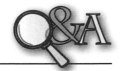

1. **B.** More common due to increased healthcare needs. Older adults suffer from comorbidities more frequently than other segments of the population. Pain may even be related to frequent healthcare-related visits and interventions.

2. **A.** Loss of subcutaneous tissue and muscle mass. Despite the fact that older adults may have gained weight throughout their lifetimes, fat deposition changes. Muscle mass decreases as a result of inactivity and hormonal changes of aging.

3. **C.** Intermittent claudication, pain resulting from changes in circulation in the lower extremities.

4. **B.** May be masked by over-the-counter medication used by the elderly to self-treat conditions ranging from headache to osteoarthritis.

5. **C.** Inability to vocalize or describe pain because of changes in mentation or loss of language abilities.

6. **C.** Changes in liver function, resulting in longer elevated serum drug levels. This may be best managed with less frequent dosing, using longer intervals between doses.

7. **A.** Careful evaluation of all medications currently in use before adding analgesics. A comprehensive medication assessment is crucial to pain management.

8. **C.** Use enteric coated tablets, if they are available. If not, taking the medication with food is a second alternative.

9. **B.** An elderly person may be more susceptible to burns because of thin, frail skin and decreased subcutaneous tissue.

10. **D.** Mentation, nutrition, and compliance are all important components of chronic pain management.

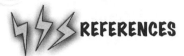

REFERENCES

Acute Pain Management Guideline Panel. (1992). *Acute pain management: operative or medical procedures and trauma. AHCPR Pub No. 92-0032.* Rockville, MD: Agency for Health Care Policy and Research, Public Health Service, U.S. Department of Health and Human Services.

American Geriatric Society Panel on Chronic Pain in Older Persons. (1998). The management of chronic pain in older persons. *J Am Geriatr Soc, 46,* 635–651.

Dworkin, R. H., Johnson, R. W., Breuer, J., et al. (2007). Recommendations for the management of herpes zoster. *Clin Infect Dis, 44* Suppl 1, S1–S26.

Gagliese, L., Katz, J., & Melzack, R. (1999). Pain in the elderly. In: P. D. Wall & R. Melzack (Eds.), *Textbook of pain* (4th ed., pp. 991–1006). Edinburgh, UK: Churchill Livingstone.

Gagliese, L., & Melzack, R. (1997). Chronic pain in elderly people. *Pain, 70*(1), 3.

Galloway, S., & Turner, L. (1999). Pain assessment in older adults who are cognitively impaired. *J Gerontol Nurs, 25*(7), 34.

Girard, N. (2000). Care of the geriatric patient. In: M. L. Phippen & M. P. Wells (Eds.), *Patient care during operative and invasive procedures* (pp. 675–695). Philadelphia: W. B. Saunders.

Herr, K., Bjoro, K., Steffensmeier, J., & Rakel, B. (2006). *Acute pain management in older adults.* Iowa City, IA: University of Iowa Gerontological Nursing Interventions Research Center, Research Translation and Dissemination Core.

Lanas, A., & Ferrandez, A. (2007). Inappropriate prevention of NSAID-induced gastrointestinal events among long-term users in the elderly. *Drugs and Aging, 24*(2), 121–131.

Pasero, C., Reed, B. A., & McCaffery, M. (1999). Pain in the elderly. In: M. McCaffery & C. Pasero (Eds.), *Pain: clinical manual for nursing practice* (2nd ed., pp. 674–710). St. Louis, MO: Mosby.

Simon, L. S., Lipman, A. G., Jacox, A. K., et al. (2002). *Pain in osteoarthritis, rheumatoid arthritis and juvenile chronic arthritis* (2nd ed.). Glenview, IL: American Pain Society.

Victor, K. (2001). Properly assessing pain in the elderly. *RN, 64*(5), 45–49.

Young, D., Mentes, J. C., & Titler, M. G. (1999). Acute pain management protocol. *J Gerontol Nurs, 26*(5), 10.

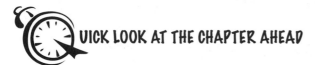

Unrelieved pain is one of the most common causes of somatic distress in the months, weeks, and days before death. Because individuals often become lethargic during the dying process, healthcare providers need to be aware of the potential for pain during this time. Patients with advanced cancer are more likely to be assessed and treated for potential pain as they near death than patients with a history of non-malignant pain. It is imperative that all patients near death are assessed and treated for pain, regardless of their diagnosis.

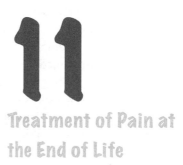

11

Treatment of Pain at the End of Life

TERMS
- ☐ ceiling effect
- ☐ Do Not Resusitate (DNR)
- ☐ epidural analgesia
- ☐ equianalgesic dose
- ☐ intrathecal analgesia
- ☐ morphine sulfate sustained release
- ☐ narcotic naïve
- ☐ neuropathic pain
- ☐ nonsteroidal anti-inflammatory drugs (NSAIDs)
- ☐ opioid
- ☐ parenteral
- ☐ prognostic indicators
- ☐ transdermal

191

CASE STUDY 1

S. B. is an 80-year-old female with stage IV breast cancer and metastasis to the bone. She is not a candidate for chemotherapy or radiation and has elected to remain at home without further treatment for her disease. She is being followed by a home hospice agency. For several months, S. B. has been taking **morphine sulfate sustained release** (MS Contin®) 90 mg orally every 12 hours and ibuprofen 200 mg orally every 8 hours to manage low back pain. She occasionally takes morphine sulfate immediate release 30 mg for breakthrough pain. Otherwise, MS Contin and ibuprofen control her pain well.

For the past 3 days, S. B. has been extremely weak and fatigued, incontinent of urine, and sleeping most of the day and night. When she is awake, she has no desire to eat. The hospice nurse informs the family that the signs and symptoms indicate that her body may be slowing down and that she is likely near death. Given this change in her clinical condition, someone in the home will need to take on the role of managing her medications so that she remains comfortable until death.

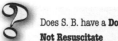 Does S. B. have a **Do Not Resuscitate (DNR)** order? Who should assume the role of medication manager in the home? How should the nurse assist this person? What might you (the nurse) establish as a plan for the medication management of S. B.'s pain? What are potential barriers to providing optimal pain management to S. B.?

CASE STUDY 2

T. C. is a 74-year-old female with severe chronic obstructive pulmonary disease (COPD), cor pulmonale, osteoporosis, and arthritis. She is dependent on home oxygen and oral steroids. Other medications include diuretics, **nonsteroidal anti-inflammatory drugs (NSAIDs),** multiple bronchodilators, and respiratory medications. She states that she wants to avoid further hospitalizations for her disease, does not want to be intubated or resuscitated, and that she has a living will and durable power of attorney for

Does T. C. have a Do Not Resuscitate order? Who should assume the role of medication manager in the home? How should the nurse assist this person? What might you (the nurse) establish as a plan for the medication management of T. C.'s pain? What are potential barriers to providing optimal pain management to T. C.?

health care in place. She is currently being followed by a registered nurse from the transitional care department of a home hospice agency.

For 5 days, T. C. has been on oral antibiotics for acute bronchitis, but her overall condition has steadily declined. Today she is lethargic, unable to stand, and having difficulty swallowing her medications. The home care nurse discusses T. C.'s condition with her, her family, and her physician, and they develop a plan of care.

 ## PAIN IN PATIENTS NEAR DEATH

The literature indicates that unrelieved pain is one of the most common causes of somatic distress in the months, weeks, and days before death. Most of what is known about symptoms in individuals near death has been derived from studies on patients with cancer. However, many individuals die from other chronic diseases that are also capable of causing pain and discomfort.

Approximately two-thirds of patients with advanced cancer have moderate to severe pain. Pain in patients with cancer may result from tumor involvement, cancer related procedures or treatment, or causes unrelated to the cancer or its treatment. Most chronic pain in people with cancer is related to tumor involvement, with bone pain and compression of neural structures the most common causes. Clients with cancer may experience pain throughout the course of their disease. In some situations, treatments such as radiation or chemotherapy can be given to reduce tumor size, resulting in a decrease in pain intensity. Medication, however, is the mainstay of treatment for chronic cancer pain, and the medication is generally given for life to prevent pain from recurring. Adjustments in medication are made if the intensity, frequency, or character of pain changes over time.

The healthcare and lay communities are familiar with the fact that cancer is often a terminal disease. Healthcare providers also demonstrate an understanding that pain occurs in clients with cancer and that analgesia for pain, especially in advanced disease, is appropriate. It is questionable, however, how often healthcare providers utilize prognostic indicators for other chronic, life-threatening diseases and how well symptoms such as pain are treated in clients with noncancer diagnoses near death.

The hospice movement has done a great deal to educate people about the process of death and dying, and the need to provide quality end-of-life care. Although the majority of clients receiving hospice services have historically had a cancer diagnosis, hospice and other palliative care services are not limited to clients with cancer. The National Hospice and Palliative Care Organization has published prognostic guidelines to help identify when individuals with chronic disease other than cancer are in the terminal phase of their disease. **Prognostic indicators** exist for renal failure, COPD, end-stage cardiac disease, amyotrophic lateral sclerosis, dementia, and acquired immunodeficiency disease (AIDS). Such indicators are not meant to emphasize the negative aspects of chronic disease. Instead, they are meant to assist healthcare providers in identifying individuals who would likely benefit from services that promote quality end-of-life care. Despite the availability of these and other measures of prognoses, they are underutilized in guiding treatment at the end of life. As a result, many individuals near the end of their lives are not provided with quality palliative care, and they risk dying in pain. Such were the findings of the 1995 Support Study, which looked at factors impacting care for hospitalized adults at the end of life. When death nears, adults with cancer are likely receiving long-acting narcotics to control severe pain. Clients without cancer are less likely to be treated for severe pain and less likely to receive narcotics, particularly long-acting formulas. Because many of these clients are **narcotic naïve** (that is, do not routinely take narcotic medications), it is likely they will not require the high doses of narcotics that clients with chronic cancer pain require. In fact, clients dying from a cause other than cancer may achieve comfort from pain with non-narcotics and nonpharmacological approaches to pain. What is imperative is that the pain is assessed and treatment is offered, regardless of the etiology. Too often, however, pain is not assessed, particularly in people who become lethargic, which often occurs prior to death. Perceived risks of medications for pain, such as respiratory depression and lethargy, also act as barriers to treatment.

 Nurses should never assume that because a person is lethargic, they are not experiencing pain.

As individuals near death, pain may increase, decrease, or remain at the same level of intensity. As death nears, however, patients may lose the ability to communicate their pain because of the lethargy, decreased level of consciousness, or cognitive impairment that often accompanies the dying process.

The risk that pain will continue or recur and the loss of ability to rely on client reports mandate that medication regimens controlling cancer pain continue to be given to dying clients until death occurs. (The exception to this is a patient with diminished hepatic and renal function with no urine output, who is receiving routine dosing or a continuous infusion of morphine. Metabolites of morphine may remain active as analgesics in the body and accumulate, risking morphine toxicity and delirium. In this case morphine may be decreased). When clients can no longer report pain, alternate methods of assessing pain need to be performed. These include assessment of nonverbal pain behaviors.

Just as decreasing or eliminating analgesic medications in a client with cancer who is near death is generally not appropriate, it is not appropriate to eliminate analgesic medications in clients near death from a nonmalignant disease. It is not always clear, however, when a client is near death, and signs and symptoms such as a decreased level of consciousness may be falsely attributed to narcotics. In situations where the etiology of a decreased level of consciousness in a client with a life-threatening illness is not clear, the nurse or physician may be tempted to decrease or withhold narcotics to assess their role in the change of mental status. The nurse or physician should know, however, that clients who have not had recent increases in their narcotics are likely tolerant to the sedating effects of narcotics, and the narcotics are probably not the cause of their change in mental status.

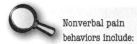

Nonverbal pain behaviors include:

- Tense body language—for example, grimacing of facial muscles; clenched fists, knees pulled up tightly.
- Frightened facial expression—for example, alarmed appearance with open eyes and pleading face.
- Noise or speech with negative quality—for example, moaning or groaning.
- Restless behavior—for example, constant jittery movement or squirming, rubbing of body parts, forceful touching, or trying to get away from hurt area.

 Caution should be taken in decreasing analgesic dosing in clients near death because of the risk of recurrent pain.

Discussion and establishment of the goals of treatment in a client with chronic disease and pain who may be near death should preclude withdrawal of analgesic medications. If the patients' goal is relief of pain, sedation or other side effects of effective medications are often acceptable Failure to provide adequate treatment to relieve pain is not.

The most notable difference in the treatment of pain at the end of life for clients with both malignant and nonmalignant disease is that patients with cancer are more likely to receive narcotics to prevent their pain, often in the long-acting form. Patients with non-malignant pain are more likely to receive non-opioid analgesics, most likely in the short-acting form.

 ## NONOPIOID ANALGESICS

Nonopioid analgesics include acetaminophen and nonsteroidal anti-inflammatory drugs (NSAIDs) such as aspirin and ibuprofen. Although often effective for mild to moderate pain of somatic or visceral origin, these drugs have a **ceiling effect** that limits the amount of the drug that can be administered safely. NSAIDs may also cause adverse effects such as gastrointestinal upset and bleeding. Although clients with rheumatoid arthritis or bone pain often benefit from NSAIDs, histories of gastrointestinal hemorrhage or a low platelet count may make these drugs a poor choice. A thorough assessment of the client's past experiences with pain and analgesics and their side effects is essential to optimal pain management. The experience of pain is somewhat individual, and using analgesics that have been effective for past pain experiences is recommended.

Pain related to advanced cancer is generally treated with narcotic analgesics. The oral route is preferred because it is relatively safe, noninvasive, and more cost effective. Medications given orally are also generally easy to administer until the patient has difficulty swallowing. Once pain is controlled, prevention of recurrent pain becomes the goal. Prevention of recurrent pain generally requires administering medication around-the-clock to maintain an adequate level of analgesia. Non-narcotics such as acetaminophen or NSAIDs are the first line of treatment for mild to moderate pain. When pain persists or increases, an **opioid** such as codeine or hydrocodone is added, often in the form of a combination drug (for example, oxycodone and acetaminophen). Although combination medications are often effective in controlling mild to moderate pain, their use is limited by the content of acetaminophen or NSAID in the medication. For example, 4 g of acetaminophen is the 24-hour limit for adults. Toxicity could occur with doses exceeding this.

Nurses must ensure that patients take no more than 4 g of acetaminophen in one 24-hour period.

OPIOID (NARCOTIC) ANALGESICS

Persistent pain or pain that is moderate to severe in intensity is generally treated by increasing the opioid potency of drugs. Pure opioid agonists such as morphine, hydromorphone, and oxycodone are the drugs of choice because they do not have a ceiling effect (that is, limited dose requirement). These pure agonists are often given in an extended-release formula to ease administration and prolong control of pain. Medications without a ceiling effect in long-acting formulas include extended-release morphine (for example, MS Contin; Oramorph) and controlled or sustained-release oxycodone (for example, Oxycontin SR).

Neuropathic pain may require adjuvant medications in addition to narcotics. Antidepressants, anticonvulsants, corticosteroids, neuroleptics, and local anesthetics in various doses can enhance analgesic efficacy in specific situations.

CHANGING ROUTES OF ADMINISTRATION NEAR DEATH

A problem with continuing analgesics until death is that clients with a decreased level of consciousness often lose the ability to safely swallow medications, particularly long-acting medications that cannot be chewed or crushed. Alternative routes and dosing schedules to replace analgesics previously taken orally need to be identified.

Assistance with finding an alternative route generally requires the input of a physician or nurse who is knowledgeable in palliative care. Access to a pharmacist who is able to advise and compound medications for alternative routes is also advantageous.

Short-acting narcotics in liquid form or as crushed tablets may be given sublingually in the buccal mucosa of the cheek or lower lip. The effectiveness of this approach in preventing pain, however, is limited by the amount of the drug that can be given at one time. Clients who have had their pain controlled with only occasional analgesics as opposed to long-acting analgesics may continue to have good control of pain with short-acting analgesics given sublingually. However, clients who have been on high doses of long-acting analgesics likely will require an additional route for administration of medications.

An appropriate alternative route for several long-acting narcotics and non-narcotics is the rectal route. Advantages of this route are that dosing requirements of certain oral medications are the same whether they are administered orally or rectally. Retaining the same dosing requirement eliminates the need to calculate equianalgesic doses and to obtain or purchase new prescriptions. Not only does a switch from oral to rectal administration save family and healthcare providers time and money, it also facilitates ongoing control of pain by avoiding major changes in the treatment plan.

 Not all analgesics can be administered rectally.

Although the rectal route is a good alternative for some dying clients, it is not a good alternative for all. Clients with loose stool, constipation, or rectal bleeding may not adequately absorb the analgesia given rectally. Clients with low platelet counts are at risk for bleeding from insertion of medication into the rectum, and clients with lesions of the anus or rectum may experience pain. Rectal administration of analgesics may also pose problems for caregivers who have assumed the responsibility of administering medications near death. Problems cited by family caregivers include aversion to touching the rectum, clients' aversion to having the rectum touched, and difficulty turning the client or inserting the medication into the rectum. It should also be noted that not all oral analgesics can be administered rectally. Assessment for potential problems related to rectal administration of a medication should be made before plans to maintain a client's control of pain are solidified.

Routes of administration of analgesics other than the rectal route are also available to control pain in dying clients with cancer or other pain-related conditions. The **transdermal** route is the least invasive alternative route. Use of this route, however, is limited by the number of available analgesics capable of providing relief through transdermal administration, particularly if the analgesia is long acting. Fentanyl is a potent narcotic analgesic that can be used in place of another long-acting oral analgesic, after the appropriate equianalgesic dose is calculated.

If pain near death escalates and cannot be adequately controlled via the oral, rectal, or transdermal route, a client may need to be switched to a continuous subcutaneous or intravenous (IV) narcotic infusion. If the client has an existing IV access (for example, central line), an intravenous infusion would be initiated. If no existing access is available, a subcutaneous infusion would be initiated.

The subcutaneous route for continuous administration of narcotics provides blood levels of opiates comparable to those achieved by the IV route. Subcutaneous access is also easier to initiate.

Changing a client from the oral route to subcutaneous or IV infusion requires calculation of the 24-hour dose of oral analgesia (controlled release and immediate release) and calculation of the equianalgesic dose for the parenteral route. An hourly rate is calculated by dividing the 24-hour total **parenteral equianalgesic dose** of drug by 24 and dividing that number by 2. Division by 2 is done when first making the change from oral to parenteral to ensure that the dose is not too potent (**Table 11-1**). Once the parenteral infusion is initiated, the dose can be titrated up as needed to control the pain. Because treatment of pain is often complex, specialists in pain management may be needed to achieve optimal control of pain. Palliative care programs such as hospice often have pain teams composed of experts in pain management who will take referrals or consult by phone. These programs also have access to pharmacists and supply companies that can quickly implement a plan of care, even at odd hours.

Clients with intractable pain who do not respond to optimal treatment using the therapies described here may require invasive interventions utilizing **intrathecal** or **epidural analgesia** with catheters, nerve blocks, neurosurgery, or surgery to relieve an obstruction of a compression that is causing pain.

CASE STUDY 1 RESOLVED

The route for S. B.'s analgesics needs to be changed from the oral route because she is weak and may have difficulty swallowing the pill, and because she should not chew a sustained-release tablet. If acceptable to the

Table 11-1   Conversion of Morphine Sulfate from Oral Route to Subcutaneous or Intravenous Route

Step 1. Calculate 24-hour dose of oral narcotic analgesia (controlled release and immediate release)
Add all MS taken in 24 hours:
Example: MS Contin, 90 mg every 12 hours
Immediate release MS, 30 mg (two doses in 24 hours)

   90 mg
   90 mg
 + 60 mg
 ─────────
  240 mg of MS (oral dose) in 24 hours

Step 2. Refer to the equianalgesic dosing chart and calculate the equianalgesic dose for the parenteral route.
Morphine:
Oral 30 mg = 10 mg parenteral

$$\frac{10 \text{ mg}}{30 \text{ mg}} = \frac{x}{240 \text{ mg}}$$

   30x = 2400 mg

    x   = 80 mg parenteral dose in 24 hours

Step 3. Divide the 24-hour parenteral dose by 2. (Many consider the parenteral dose on the equianalgesic chart equivalent to an intramuscular dose.)

   80 ÷ 2 = 40 mg IV or SC in 24 hours

Step 4. Calculate the hourly rate (SC/IV dose) by dividing the 24-hour IV dose by 24.

   40 mg ÷ 24 = 1.66 mg each hour, or 2 mg each hour

MS = morphine sulfate; IV = intravenous; SC = subcutaneous

client and family, the MSSR can be given rectally, beginning with the same dose as that given orally (90 mg every 12 hours). MSIR must also be made available to administer for breakthrough pain. The liquid form of MSIR, which peaks in 30 minutes, is often preferred over MSIR tablets because it is concentrated and a small amount of fluid can provide substantial analgesia (1 mL = 20 mg; 0.25 mL = 5 mg). Liquid MSIR can be given orally or sublingually in the cheeks. If S. B. were converted from MSIR tablets to MSIR liquid, she would receive 1.5 mL of liquid (20 mg/mL) to equal the 30 mg dose she previously received for breakthrough pain. However, if cost is an issue, the MSIR in tablet form could be given rectally or could be crushed and given sublingually for breakthrough pain. To substitute ibuprofen tablets, liquid or suppository forms of an equivalent NSAID may be used. Continuing the ibuprofen may be important if it is being given for pain related to bone metastasis.

CASE STUDY 2 RESOLVED

Although T. C. does not have cancer, she has COPD with cor pulmonale, which indicates advanced disease. She has been receiving NSAIDs, most likely for pain related to her arthritis and osteoporosis, but is no longer able to swallow her medications. A liquid or suppository form of ibuprofen could be tried. Her respiratory status continues to be managed by inhalation with the appropriate bronchodilators. However, nebulization of these bronchodilators with a mask may be required for optimal absorption of the medication. A small dose of liquid morphine (5 mg = 0.25 mL of a 20 mg/mL concentration) can also be administered to help treat pain or control dyspnea that T. C. is likely to experience. It should be noted that T. C. is narcotic naïve (that is, she has not been taking narcotics routinely). Thus, she should be started on no more than 5 mg of MSIR orally or sublingually at one time.

 ## SUMMARY

Pain is a common symptom of disease in clients who are near death, regardless of the cause. All healthcare providers should prioritize the assessment and optimal treatment of pain in clients near death. Treatment generally requires nonopioid or opioid analgesics to prevent the recurrence of known pain and treat escalation or new occurrences. To ensure optimal comfort near death, healthcare providers must be knowledgeable about alternative routes for analgesia, analgesic dosing, and multiple other issues related to pain near death, or make appropriate and timely referrals to palliative care providers with expertise in the management of pain.

The treatment of pain suggested for the two clients in the case studies is intended to provide an example of a common analgesic plan of care at the end of life. It should be noted, however, that the treatment of pain at the end of life is often complex and optimally involves a more comprehensive assessment, individualized plan of care, and ongoing evaluation of the pain and distress.

CASE STUDY QUESTIONS

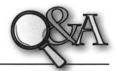

1. Identify differences and similarities between the cases of S. B. and T. C.

2. Would T. C. require a cancer diagnosis to be admitted on a hospice benefit?

3. Given the information provided, what would you identify as a priority of care for S. B. and T. C.?

4. Given S. B. and T. C.'s difficulty swallowing, what must the nurse do to permit continued pain relief?

CASE STUDY ANSWERS

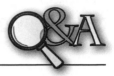

1. S. B. is a client in hospice, which generally indicates a life expectancy of 6 months or less. S. B. has a malignant disease in advanced stages. T. C. is a client in transitional care. We know nothing about her prognosis, but cor pulmonale is a life-threatening disease.

   S. B's symptoms include lower back pain, which has been well controlled with oral extended-release morphine, ibuprofen, and immediate-release morphine as needed. T. C's symptoms are not well defined in the case, but she takes NSAIDS most likely for pain related to her arthritis and osteoporosis.

   S. B's symptoms of extreme weakness and fatigue, sleeping incontinence, and anorexia may indicate that she is actively dying. T. C. has acute bronchitis, which is life-threatening to a person with COPD and cor pulmonale. Her lethargy, inability to stand, and difficulty swallowing indicate she is not improving and possibly declining.

   S. B. is a client in hospice, which indicates that she elected to avoid further hospitalization (unless the situation changes) and that someone has likely taken the responsibility of being a primary caregiver. S. B. may or may not have agreed to DNR (do not resuscitate) status, depending on the policy of the particular hospice with which she has contracted. T. C. is not a client in hospice, but she wants to avoid further hospitalizations and she is a DNR.

2. No. Although the majority of clients receiving hospice services have traditionally had a cancer diagnosis, hospice is not limited to clients with cancer. Prognostic indicators also exist for COPD.

3. A priority of care for S. B. and T. C. is comfort (for example, control of pain).

4. The nurse must arrange to have appropriate analgesics and other medications for symptoms of distress in the home, which can be given easily to clients who are unable to swallow. S. B. will need to be continued on her MSSR, which can be given rectally. Her MSIR may be given safely in the buccal mucosa, rectally, or transdermally in gel form.

   T. C. may receive ibuprofen in suppository form or in a gel if compounding facilities are available.

CHAPTER 11 • REVIEW QUESTIONS

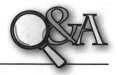

1.　Which of the following statements about pain near the end of life is accurate?
    A.　Pain near death increases only in clients with cancer
    B.　Pain is generally not present in the noncancer population
    C.　Pain at the end of life is extremely difficult to treat
    D.　Pain may increase, decrease, or remain the same as death nears

2.　Of the following, which analgesic is limited in terms of the dose that can be administered?
    A.　Acetaminophen
    B.　Methadone
    C.　Morphine sulfate
    D.　Oxycontin SR

3.　The preferred route for administration of analgesics in a client with mild to moderate pain is:
    A.　Intravenous
    B.　Oral
    C.　Rectal
    D.　Transdermal

4.　For 3 months John has been receiving Duragesic (fentanyl transdermal system) 50 µg for pain related to carcinoma of the lung. John becomes obtunded, difficult to arouse, and is thought to be near death. The nurse should:
    A.　Remove the Duragesic patch
    B.　Discontinue changing Duragesic patches
    C.　Contact the physician
    D.　Continue the Duragesic as ordered

5.　Which of the following statements about prognostic indicators is accurate:
    A.　They are meant to be used only for clients with malignant disease
    B.　They assist in identifying individuals who could benefit from end-of-life care
    C.　They have no impact on the treatment of pain at the end of life
    D.　They have been well-utilized within our healthcare system

6. Mrs. Jones has been taking MS Contin 60 mg orally every 12 hours for pain related to breast cancer. She has been declining and can no longer swallow. Which of the following interventions is most appropriate:

    A.   Start IV morphine at an equianalgesic dose
    B.   Start subcutaneous morphine at an equianalgesic dose
    C.   Rectal administration of MS Contin
    D.   Discontinue MS Contin

ANSWERS AND RATIONALES

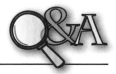

1. **D.** Pain may occur in any client near death. Early and ongoing treatment of pain plays a large role in preventing severe pain from occurring at the end of life. The intensity of pre-existing pain may remain the same, may increase, or may decrease as death nears.

2. **A.** Four grams of acetaminophen is the 24-hour limit for adults. Toxicity could occur with doses exceeding this.

3. **B.** Oral route is preferred because it is noninvasive, relatively safe, easily titrated, easily administered, and relatively inexpensive. Severe pain that does not respond to oral analgesia may require IV analgesics to obtain good pain control.

4. **D.** A decreased level of consciousness is a common manifestation of dying. With a sudden decrease in a client's level of consciousness, healthcare providers may be tempted to decrease or discontinue narcotics in order to evaluate their possible role in the change in mental status. If there has been no recent increase in narcotic and the client is declining from disease, narcotics are not likely the cause of the mental status change, and they should not be discontinued.

5. **B.** Prognostic indicators have been underutilized. When used, they assist in identifying those who would benefit from quality end-of-life care.

6. **C.** The rectal route is a good alternative for administration of some long-acting narcotics such as morphine sulfate extended release (for example, MS Contin). The same dose ordered orally can be given rectally, thus eliminating the need to calculate an equianalgesic dose and obtain a different medication. An IV infusion may be appropriate if the client has existing IV access. However, this would require obtaining a new prescription, the medication for IV administration, and appropriate equipment. A less invasive route, such as rectal or transdermal, is generally preferred when clients can no longer swallow.

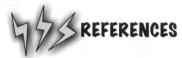

REFERENCES

Coyle, N., & Goldstein, M. L. (2006). Pain assessment and pharmacological interventions. In: M. L. Matzo & D. W. Sherman (Eds.), *Palliative care nursing: quality care at the end of life* (2nd ed., pp. 345–405). New York: Springer.

Emanuel, L., Ferris, F.D., von Gunten, C.F. & Von Roenn, J. (2006). The Last Hours of Living: Practical Advice for Clinicians. *Medscape.* www.medscapte .com/viewarticle.

Feldt, K. (2000). Checklist of nonverbal pain indicators. *Pain Mgt Nursing*, 1, 13–21.

Foley, K. M. (2004). Acute and chronic pain syndromes. In D. Doyle, G. H. Hanks, N. Cherny, & K. Calman (Eds.), *Oxford textbook of palliative medicine* (3rd ed., pp. 298–316). Oxford, UK: Oxford University Press.

Gavrin, J., & Chapman, R. (1995). Clinical management of dying patients. *Western J Med*, *163*, 268–277.

Hospice Pharmacia. (2006). *The Hospice Pharmacia Medication Use Guidelines.* (8th. ed.). www.hospicepharmacia.com.

Management of Cancer Guideline Panel (1994). *Management of cancer pain clinical practice guidelines. AHCPR Pub No. 94-0592.* Rockville, MD: Agency for Health Care Policy and Research, Public Health Services, U.S. Department of Health and Human Services.

National Comprehensive Cancer Network, *NCCN adult cancer pain clinical practice guidelines in oncology, v.1.2007.* Retrieved July 31, 2007 from www. nccn.org.

National Hospice Organization (1996). *Medical guidelines for determining prognosis in selected non-cancer diseases.* (2nd ed.). Arlington, VA: Author.

Paice, J. A., & Fine, P. G. (2001). Pain at the end of life. In: B. R. Ferrell & N. Coyle (Eds.). *Textbook of palliative nursing* (pp. 76–90). Oxford, UK: Oxford University Press.

St. Marie, B., & Loeb, J. L. (2002). Gerontologic pain management. In B. St. Marie (Ed.), *Core curriculum for pain management nursing* (pp. 417–426). Philadelphia: W.B. Saunders.

Support Study Principal Investigators. (1995). A controlled trial to improve care for seriously ill hospitalized patients: the study to understand prognoses and preferences for outcomes and risks of treatments (support). *JAMA*, *274*(20), 1591–1598.

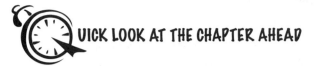

When treating a person's pain, the prescriber (physician or nurse practitioner) should take into account the presumed cause of the pain, and ensure that the treatment will be feasible and effective. In discharging a patient from a facility to home it is the responsibility of the nurse to facilitate the implementation of the plan. Referral of the patient to providers who will not be seeing them for hours or days after discharge does not relieve the prescriber of providing the patient with adequate pain relief.

Treating acute surgical pain, which is supposed to decrease with time, is different from treating malignant pain, which is likely to increase. Although providers may not have recent experience treating malignant pain, they are still mandated to, ensure adequate pain control for patients, regardless of where the person is (that is, hospital or home). Nurses need to be aware of the many barriers there are within our health-care system, to ensure adequate pain control for all patients, throughout the healthcare continuum.

12

The Variable
Treatment of Pain

TERMS
- □ around-the-clock
- □ continuous dosing
- □ continuous infusion
- □ demand bolus
- □ demand dose
- □ lockout interval
- □ parenteral
- □ patient controlled analgesia (PCA)

209

CASE STUDY

J. D. is a 34-year-old male who was admitted to the hospital for abdominal pain to rule out peptic ulcer disease. During a diagnostic work-up, a biopsy was taken from tissue in the stomach via esophagogastroduodenoscopy (EGD). The biopsy was found positive for gastric adenocarcinoma. J. D. underwent surgical resection of the stomach under general anesthesia, but the tumor was not completely resected. Postoperatively, J. D. was prescribed morphine sulfate 1 mg intravenously (IV) via demand mode of a **patient-controlled analgesia (PCA)** pump with a **lockout interval** of 6 minutes and a 4-hour maximum limit of 30 mg.

On the first postoperative night, J. D. rated his abdominal pain as 7 on a scale of 0 to 10 (0 = no pain; 10 = worst pain ever), after receiving 8 mg (that is, eight doses of 1 mg each) of morphine for two consecutive hours.

Recognizing that the patient's pain was not optimally controlled with near-maximum **demand doses**, the nurse contacted the surgeon to request an increase in opioid analgesia. The surgeon ordered the morphine to be given via the **continuous mode**, in addition to the demand mode. The dose for the continuous mode is ordered to be 2 mg to 3 mg/hour, and the demand bolus doses are increased to 1.5 mg every 6 minutes, with a 4 hour maximum of 40mg. Within an hour, the patient reported that his pain decreased to a level of 3 using 8 boluses. The patient is sleeping in naps, but easily arousable and oriented when awake, with a respiratory rate of 16 both during sleep and when awake. Within 2 hours the client rates his pain level "0," receiving a continuous hourly rate of 2 mg, with two demand doses each hour.

What is the nurse's priority intervention at this time? What should be the goal for J. D.'s pain on the first postoperative night?

Continuous infusion of a low-dose of opioid (for example, morphine sulfate 1–2 mg/hour) is designed to maintain the serum opioid level to provide a balanced level of analgesia. Demand doses, which are delivered when the patient pushes a bolus button, are used for breakthrough pain.

Continuous infusions and/or frequent **demand boluses** are more likely to lead to accumulation of the opioid in the serum, with subsequent side effects. Life threatening side effects include respiratory depression and a decrease in level of consciousness. Protocols to routinely monitor for signs and symptoms of side effects and opioid accumulation must be followed by the nurse caring for the patient.

On the third postoperative day, the surgeon orders a decrease in the continuous dose of morphine to 1 mg each hour, with a decrease in the bolus to 0.5 mg every 6 minutes as needed (PRN). The patient states that his pain at times is at "5," usually after activity, but decreases to "0" quickly with demand doses. He continues to receive an hourly continuous infusion and occasional demand doses of morphine for another 3 days. On the sixth day after surgery, the surgeon discontinues the intravenous (IV) morphine via the PCA, and orders oxycodone 5 mg/acetaminophen 325 mg, one to two tablets every 4 hours PRN for pain. The patient is discharged home, but no prescription is written for analgesia after discharge. Discharge orders do, however, include an order for an IV antibiotic to be infused at 8:00 AM daily by a home-health nurse. Arrangements are also made for the client to see a medical oncologist 1 week after discharge for possible treatment of his grade III gastric cancer.

J. D. receives two tablets of oxycodone 5 mg/acetaminophen 325 mg (Percocet) in the hospital and is discharged home at 4:30 PM. By 9:00 PM, J. D. has severe abdominal pain. J. D.'s wife first calls the surgeon to report the client's severe pain, and the surgeon instructs her to give two tablets of acetaminophen every 4 hours PRN. J. D. receives no relief from the acetaminophen, and his wife contacts the on-call home-health agency.

Because of his diagnosis of advanced gastric cancer, J. D. is admitted to the transitional care/hospice department of the home-health agency. Nurses in this department have intensive training in management of pain and embrace the philosophy that pain should be aggressively treated and controlled, particularly with advanced disease. Recognizing that the surgeon did not arrange for analgesia after discharge, the on-call transitional care nurse contacts the medical oncologist with whom J. D. has an appointment the following week. Although the oncologist states that he generally does not order medication when he has not yet seen the patient, he agrees to order it at this time based on the data provided by the nurse. The nurse instructs the doctor to call the hospice pharmacy, because she

 How much pain would be expected for J. D. on his day of discharge? What should have been the goal for J. D. after discharge? What could have been done by the nurse to have facilitated better pain control? How should the home-health nurse assist J. D.?

Why was J. D. discharged home without a prescription for an analgesia? How could this have been avoided? What are the barriers in health care related to adequate pain relief?

knows that the pharmacist there will fill a narcotic with a telephone order from the physician. The oncologist orders morphine sulfate 20 mg/mL, the dose to be 10 to 20 mg orally (PO) PRN every 1 to 2 hours.

 In an effort to prevent the diversion of opioids from patients in pain to people abusing them, the Drug Enforcement Administration of the U.S. government and State Boards of Pharmacies regulate the prescription of narcotics. Specific laws vary among the states, but pharmacists often are not able to fill prescriptions for narcotic analgesics without a written prescription.

UNDERTREATMENT OF PAIN

In the 1990s, lack of standardization and ineffective pain management prompted the federal government to develop and publish clinical practice guidelines on acute pain (1992) and cancer pain (1994). In 2001, the Joint Commission Accreditation of Health Care Organizations (JCAHO) published pain management standards, which were meant to ensure that pain was being assessed at regular intervals and managed appropriately. Despite these guidelines and standards, pain continues to be inadequately managed due to insufficient knowledge of the pharmacology of analgesics, healthcare provider misconceptions about potent narcotics, and fear of addiction. Some of the variability in management of pain seems to be related to the different philosophies of pain management in different practice areas.

Management of Acute/Postoperative Pain

The *Acute Pain Management Guidelines* (1992) emphasize the importance of using an adequate amount of the appropriate analgesia at the appropriate frequency to allow for prolonged analgesia. For the first 48 to 72 hours after most types of major surgery, patients typically require parenteral (that is, intravenous, epidural, or intramuscular) narcotics to obtain adequate control of pain. **Around-the-clock** dosing of these opiates are recommended (as opposed to PRN) during the first 24 to 36 hours, with the rationale that pain will be better controlled if analgesia is achieved and the therapeutic level of the drug is maintained.

As the client's pain decreases, the analgesia can be decreased. After 48 hours, many clients may be switched to oral medications, which are often less potent. Surgery-related postoperative pain should steadily decline 5 to 7 days after surgery, but analgesia with narcotics may be needed for 2 to 3 weeks after surgery for incisional pain. Pain persisting longer than 3 weeks after surgery may indicate a complication of psychological factors that need attention.

Ineffective control of postoperative pain commonly occurs when healthcare providers switch a client from **parenteral** narcotics to oral narcotics, which generally are not as potent. Ineffective control of pain also occurs when oral opioids are ordered at a frequency that does not relate to their duration of action (for example, medication with analgesic duration of 3 hours is ordered every 4 hours PRN).

CASE STUDY REVISITED

In the case of J. D., his postoperative pain was somewhat responsive to morphine but not adequately controlled with the initial dose given via the demand mode of a PCA pump. With the addition of continuous morphine and the increase in the dose of the PRN medication (from 1 mg to 1.5 mg) the patient had better pain control within 2 hours. When the continuous dose of morphine was decreased from 2 mg to 1 mg an hour on the third postoperative day, the client continued to have good control of pain. Although at times he rated his pain a 5, it generally occurred with activity, and the pain continued to be quickly relieved with demand doses of morphine. Thus, J. D.'s pain seemed to be managed adequately until the sixth postoperative day, when the continuous and demand doses were abruptly discontinued. Although an oral narcotic was ordered, it was not as potent as the medication J. D. had been receiving, and it was not continued after discharge.

Preparing for Postoperative Discharge

To prepare postoperative clients for discharge, parenteral medications are commonly switched to oral medications because the route is more convenient for self-management after discharge.

It is generally expected that both pain and analgesia will decrease as postoperative clients recover. This may also be the expectation for other clients in the acute care setting who have not undergone surgery. This should not, however, be the expected outcome for every client.

A client who has been receiving only an occasional dose of IV or intramuscular (IM) morphine may tolerate a change to an oral narcotic (thus, a decrease in potency of the dose). A client requiring IM or IV doses of morphine every 3 hours will not likely tolerate a change to oral narcotics unless the change is equal in terms of analgesic potency. For example, 10 mg of morphine sulfate given IM is equivalent to 30 mg of oral morphine. Therefore, if a client required eight doses of morphine at 10 mg IM over a 24-hour period of time (that is, every 3 hours), any equivalent less than 30 mg of oral morphine every 3 hours would be a decrease in analgesia.

Practitioners in acute care do not routinely order an equianalgesic dose of narcotics when switching routes for a postoperative patient. More typically, an oral narcotic such as 5 to 10 mg of oxycodone (with or without acetaminophen) is ordered. Many postoperative clients tolerate the change in dose well, particularly when the narcotic is combined with a non-narcotic analgesic such as acetaminophen (for example, Percocet or Tylox). Clients with severe pain will not, however, tolerate the change.

CASE STUDY REVISITED

From the third to the sixth postoperative day, J. D. received a continuous dose of 1 mg of intravenous morphine sulfate hourly, with demand doses of 0.5 mg approximately twice each shift (six times in 24 hours). The total amount of morphine he received each of these days was 27 mg intravenously. A dose of 27 mg intravenous morphine is equivalent to three times that amount (81 mg) orally. When the route of J. D.'s morphine was changed, he could have received up to 60 mg oxycodone (equivalent to 20 mg morphine and 3750 mg acetaminophen PRN) in 24 hours. He was in the hospital, however, only long enough to receive one dose (10 mg oxycodone/625 mg acetaminophen) before being discharged home. The initial change in route and decrease in analgesia may have been appropriate if J. D. had remained hospitalized with ready access to more potent opioids for back-up. However, it is inappropriate to discharge a client who has been having pain from an advanced, unresectable gastric tumor, without pain medication.

Development of a Discharge Pain Management Program

As described in the case study, J. D. developed severe abdominal pain on the first night after discharge from the hospital. When the transitional care nurse is called about his pain, she notes that J. D.'s plan of discharge did not include even a mild narcotic, and she questions why this was not done. The nurse notes that J. D. has a diagnosis of advanced gastric cancer and that he has been referred to the transitional care department of home care, which commonly follows clients with advanced malignant disease. The nurse also notes that 24 hours prior to discharge, the client required parenteral narcotics to control his pain but now has no narcotics ordered. Additionally, she notes that J. D. has a documented history of drug abuse. The transitional care nurse knows that J. D.'s pain is severe, and it will require a strong narcotic for relief. The documented history of drug abuse cues her to consider that J. D. may require a higher dose of narcotics to relieve his pain.

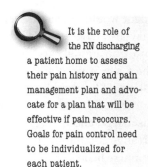 It is the role of the RN discharging a patient home to assess their pain history and pain management plan and advocate for a plan that will be effective if pain reoccurs. Goals for pain control need to be individualized for each patient.

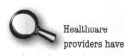 To withhold appropriate pain relief from a person with current or past addictive disease is a form of discrimination, and it is unethical. All patients deserve the best possible pain relief that may safely be provided.

Pain of malignant origin is not likely to decrease, and it needs to be treated aggressively—often chronically. If the surgeon had questions about the etiology and treatment of the pain, he should have consulted an oncologist prior to the patient's discharge.

Another factor that might have played a role in an inadequate discharge plan was J. D.'s history of drug abuse. Unlike the home health/transitional care nurse, who saw the client's history as a reason to provide adequate (and possibly higher than usual) doses of analgesia in the Case Study, practitioners in acute care often view a history of drug abuse as a reason to withhold narcotics, because of the risk of addiction. In some states, physicians must report narcotic prescriptions to known drug abusers to the federal authorities.

It is possible that a surgeon and the nurse discharging the client home believed that the

Healthcare providers have been shown to be reticent to provide opioid analgesia for patients with a current or remote history of addiction. Providers are reticent because they want to avoid inducing addiction and avoid scrutiny from the Drug Enforcement Administration (DEA), the agency that monitors the prescribing practices of healthcare providers.

client would not have severe pain after discharge. The surgeon and nurse may also have assumed that other practitioners, such as the oncologist and transitional care nurse, would manage the client's pain. Indeed, in the Case Study, the transitional care nurse's involvement led to a resolution. However, physicians and nurses in acute care should know that home healthcare nurses routinely do not see patients until the day after discharge, and that it may take days to weeks before patients are able to arrange appointments with physicians following discharge. If a physician or nurse believes that other practitioners will manage a client's pain, they should take into account the fact that there may be a period of time before the client will be seen by other healthcare professionals.

Once patients are discharged from the hospital, they are physically removed from easy contact with healthcare providers. They are often reluctant to bother physicians by phone because of fear of being perceived as complainers. Clients also may have difficulty reaching healthcare providers. For these reasons clients often avoid trying to contact physicians, even when they are in pain. Once clients do contact their providers, they first must hope the provider will respond appropriately, then must wait for the provider to call in a prescription to a pharmacy (if the pharmacy will accept a telephone order) or write a prescription. The need for a written prescription will require that it be picked up and transported to a pharmacy that stocks the medication. Clients will then need to wait until the prescription is filled. Another barrier to the treatment of pain for patients out of the hospital is the third-party payment system for prescription drugs. Many insurance providers require that medications be purchased only in those pharmacies with which they have contracted. A pharmacy that is willing to accept a telephone order may not accept the clients' medication card, may not be convenient for the family, or may have limited hours of operation.

All of these barriers can prolong pain, which when left untreated often escalates to a level at which it is difficult to relieve. The negative impact of these barriers on the treatment of pain cannot be overstated, and every effort should be taken to avoid putting a client in such a situation. Healthcare providers in both acute care and outpatient or chronic care settings should do everything they can to ensure that a client at risk for having pain has a workable plan in place, which at the very least includes access to effective analgesia. In this age of managed care, where so many clients are sick but staying in their homes, and where visits to emergency departments are discouraged (or are not approved), both nurses and physicians must look upstream, planning for what may occur when the client is home. Potential problems such as pain also need to be treated as priorities.

CASE STUDY RESOLVED

J. D. did not have ready access to effective analgesia after discharge from acute care. However, because the home transitional care nurse contacted an oncologist willing to treat J. D.'s pain, he eventually got effective treatment and relief. The resolution of J. D.'s pain occurred primarily because the home health/transitional care nurse prioritized the need to treat the client's pain promptly and did not allow any barriers to block this intervention. It was the nurse who recognized that J. D.'s pain was severe and immediately implemented a plan of care to obtain the appropriate medication promptly, despite the fact that it was midnight. The nurse knew what medication would likely relieve the client's pain safely yet promptly, knew what medications could be safely given in the home, and knew a pharmacist who could accept an emergency phone order for opioids and fill the order immediately. The nurse then went to the client's home to assist him and his family with administration of the medication, and instructed them on use of the medication to keep the pain adequately controlled.

The philosophy of palliative care is to prioritize clients' comfort and manage symptoms. Nurses working in transitional/hospice care are knowledgeable in palliative care, and they recognize that poor pain relief and symptom management is a problem. The agency where this transitional care nurse worked had a plan in place to address situations such as J. D.'s. But the key to success was not only in the plan—the key to J. D.'s relief of pain was also a result of the nurse's perception of the pain as unacceptable, and her commitment to facilitating prompt pain relief and control.

The oncologist ordered morphine sulfate elixir 20 mg/mol PO every 1 to 2 hours PRN for pain. Prior to receiving a dose, J. D. rated his pain 10 on a scale of 0–10. The nurse administered the elixir in increments of 5 to 10 mg every 10 minutes, for a total of two doses (20 mg). Although the nurse monitored the client's respiratory rate and level of sedation, she knew that the client recently had tolerated continuous and demand doses of IV morphine, which is at least three times as potent as oral morphine. As expected, J. D. tolerated 20 mg of oral morphine given over 15 minutes well, and his pain decreased to a level of 5. Within 2 hours, after receiving a total of 40 mg of oral morphine, the client rated his pain as 1 to 2 and stated he was comfortable.

Recognizing that the client's pain would likely return without long-acting or continuous morphine, the nurse instructed the client to begin taking 5 to 10 mg of morphine every 2 hours, up to 20 mg every hour if needed. The nurse arranged for the day nurse to visit the client at 8 AM to reassess his pain, evaluate the medication treatment plan, and contact the physician about implementing a long-acting analgesic if the pain was expected to continue. J. D. and his family were also instructed and encouraged to call the home-healthcare agency and request the transitional care department, if his pain was not well managed.

CHAPTER 12 · REVIEW QUESTIONS

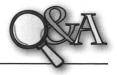

1. Lack of effective pain control is attributed to all of the following *except*:
   A. Fear of addiction
   B. Insufficient knowledge of analgesic pharmacology
   C. Misconceptions about potent narcotics
   D. The Agency for Health Care Policy and Research

2. According to AHPCR clinical practice guidelines for acute pain, for the first 24 to 36 hours postoperatively, clients should receive analgesics:
   A. Around-the-clock
   B. Orally
   C. PRN (as needed)
   D. Parenterally

3. Which of the following would be an equianalgesic dose for 10 mg of intramuscular morphine?
   A. Morphine sulfate 10 mg tablet
   B. Morphine sulfate 30 mg tablet
   C. Morphine sulfate 30 mg tablet SC
   D. Morphine sulfate 30 mg tablet IV

4. When a postoperative client's analgesics are changed from the parenteral to the oral route, the dose is usually:
   A. Decreased
   B. Increased
   C. Kept the same
   D. Determined by the patient's needs

5. M.J. is 5 days post total hip replacement. Her pain is well-controlled with MS 10 mg IM every 4 hours. Her physician elects to discontinue the parenteral morphine. Which of the following is the best plan of care for M.J.?
   A. A non-narcotic oral analgesic PRN (as needed)
   B. Around-the-clock narcotic oral analgesia, a scheduled non-narcotic oral analgesic, and parenteral narcotics as back-up
   C. Narcotic oral analgesia PRN
   D. Scheduled oral steroids

ANSWERS AND RATIONALES

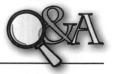

1. **D.** The AHCPR developed clinical practice guidelines for acute pain and cancer pain. These guidelines have led to improvements in pain control.

2. **A.** Pain will be better controlled if a therapeutic level of analgesia is maintained.

3. **B.** Analgesics given intramuscularly or intravenously are generally more potent than analgesics given orally. Morphine sulfate 30 mg PO would be equivalent to 10 mg morphine intramuscularly.

4. **A.** Practitioners in acute care do not routinely order an equianalgesic dose of narcotics in postoperative clients when switching from parenteral to oral routes. The rationale behind this is that incisional/surgical pain is expected to decrease over time. Back-up doses of parenteral analgesics are often ordered PRN if the oral medication does not relieve the pain.

5. **B.** A client requiring parenteral narcotics every 4 hours will not likely tolerate a change to oral analgesics. Addition of a non-narcotic will likely help, but the oral narcotics should also be given around-the-clock with parenteral narcotics used as back-up.

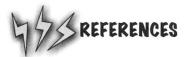# REFERENCES

Acute Pain Management Guideline Panel. (1992). *Acute pain management: operative or medical procedures and trauma clinical practice guideline. AHCPR Pub No. 92-0032.* Rockville, MD: Agency for Health Care Policy and Research, Public Health Service, U.S. Department of Health and Human Services.

American Pain Society. (1999). *Principles of analgesic use in the treatment of acute pain and cancer pain* (4th ed.). Glenview, IL: Author.

Ferrell, B., McCaffery, M., & Rhiner, M. (1992). Pain and addiction: an urgent need for change in nursing education. *J Pain Symptom Mgt, 7,* 48–55.

Joint Commission on Accreditation of Health Care Organizations. (2001). *Accreditation manual for hospitals.* Oakbrook Terrace, IL: JCAHO.

Management of Cancer Pain Guideline Panel. (1994). *Management of cancer pain: clinical practice guidelines. AHCPR Pub No. 94-0592.* Rockville, MD: Agency for Health Care Policy and Research, Public Health Service, U.S. Department of Health and Human Services.

McCaffery, M., & Ferrell, B. R. (1997). Nurses' knowledge of pain assessment and management: how much progress have we made? *J Pain Symptom Mgt, 14,* 175–188.

McCaffery, M., & Pasero, C. (1999). *Pain clinical manual* (2nd ed.). St. Louis, MO: Mosby.

Rothley, B. B., & Therrien, S. R. (2002). Acute Pain Management. In B. St. Marie (Ed.), *Core curriculum for pain management nursing* (pp. 239–272). Philadelphia: W.B. Saunders.

QUICK LOOK AT THE CHAPTER AHEAD

Individuals near death are at risk for symptoms of distress such as pain, dyspnea, agitation, nausea and vomiting. Efforts to identify and effectively treat these symptoms are essential if suffering near death is to be prevented. When clients are at home, family caregivers are expected to recognize and treat these symptoms. Though they are not professional health providers, research has shown that family caregivers are able to manage symptoms near death, with the appropriate information and ongoing clinical support from experts in palliative care.

13

Strategies to Assist Family Caregivers Treating Pain and Suffering at the End of Life

TERMS

- ☐ antiemetic
- ☐ ABH (Ativan/Benadryl/Haldol)
- ☐ buccal mucosa
- ☐ compounded
- ☐ delirium
- ☐ diphenhydramine
- ☐ dyspnea
- ☐ haloperidol
- ☐ lorazepam
- ☐ prochlorperazine
- ☐ per rectum (PR)
- ☐ symptom relief kit
- ☐ terminal agitation

CASE STUDY

M. B. is a 40-year-old woman with advanced lung cancer whose tumor has not responded to recent chemotherapy and whose overall condition is declining. When told of her condition, she requests to go home to die. A referral to home hospice is made. The hospice nurse makes the first home visit on a Friday afternoon at 4:00 PM. The nurse finds M. B. to be extremely lethargic with cool, clammy skin, all of which are manifestations of physiologic changes that occur in the last hours and days of life. M. B. is awake enough to answer simple questions and admits to pain and nausea. She is moaning at rest, and she grimaces with movement. At the start of the visit, M. B.'s mother is the only person in the house. She tells the nurse that she gave 2 tablets oxycodone/acetaminophen (Percocet) to her daughter for pain. The mother states she is able to identify all of her medications, including the **prochlorperazine** (Compazine) suppositories ordered for nausea and the morphine sulfate elixir (20 mg/mL) ordered for pain or shortness of breath (**dyspnea**).

M. B.'s husband enters the room but stands in the back, away from the client and the nurse. He has tears in his eyes and appears stunned. The nurse tells M. B's mother and husband that M. B. should not have pain, moaning, grimacing, or nausea. The nurse suggests that she administer an **antiemetic** suppository **per rectum (PR)** for the nausea, and morphine sulfate elixir by mouth for pain. With the approval of the family, the nurse administers a 25 mg suppository of prochlorperazine and 0.5 mL of a 20mg/mL (10 mg) of morphine sulfate elixir orally. Within 25 minutes, M. B. states her nausea has improved and her pain is gone, and she no longer has moaning at rest. Recognizing that M. B. will require symptom management after she leaves, the hospice nurse offers to develop a medication plan to prevent recurrent pain and nausea and to plan for treatment of other symptoms that could occur. M. B.'s mother collaborates in the plan but states that she will only be available during the day. M. B.'s husband admits he'll be in the home when

 What should the nurse do about Mr. B's perceived inability to administer medications? Identify two priority symptoms (other than pain and nausea) for which the hospice nurse would assess M. B. How does the nurse instruct family caregivers to assess M. B. for pain? How will the nurse evaluate the effectiveness of the medication management plan? What is one strategy that home hospice nurses can use to assist family caregivers with medication management of commonly occurring symptoms?

his mother-in-law leaves, listens to the nurse's recommendations for medication, but says, "I don't think I can do this."

FAMILY CAREGIVERS

With the shift in healthcare delivery from the hospital to the home and the availability of home hospice services, more clients are being cared for in the home near the end of life. Although home hospice nurses case-manage the care of clients, time spent by the nurse in the home is limited by third-party payment systems. The hospice nurse performs assessments on clients and family and collaborates with the patient, family, and hospice team to develop a plan of care to manage symptoms of distress. Symptoms present when the nurse is in the home, are often treated by the nurse. But it is the role of family caregivers to continue with the plan of care (that is, give medications) and to treat recurrent symptoms of distress.

Treating symptoms of distress requires family caregivers to recognize symptoms, identify the appropriate treatment, and administer the medication by oral, sublingual, transdermal, rectal, or intravenous route. Any one component of this process can be unfamiliar and anxiety-provoking to a lay person. And symptoms of decline that often occur near death add to the complexity of the process and the anxiety of the caregiver.

Families vary in how they organize and provide care. However, most have one person who assumes the role. Because the role involves a 24-hour-a-day commitment, others will need to assist. The majority of primary caregivers in the home have traditionally been women. The trend, however, is that males are increasingly taking on the caregiver role.

Skills to make decisions about management of symptoms are not inherent in lay caregivers. Although instructions on symptom management can be taught, lay caregivers lack the clinical judgment that healthcare professionals have acquired through education and experience to assess and treat symptoms of distress. Lay caregivers may not recognize symptoms of distress or, if able to identify symptoms, they may be reluctant to give medication to treat symptoms. Reluctance to give medication can occur for a variety of reasons. Studies have shown that caregivers have difficulty making decisions about the management of pain in clients in the home both before the terminal phase and near the client's death. Difficulties arise when clients can no longer verbally report their symptoms or collaborate on decisions to treat; when caregivers perceive that the client would prefer to defer taking treatment for a symptom; and when family members object to treatment of a symptom, administration of a certain medication such as morphine, or the use of a particular route such as the rectal route. Another barrier to caregiver treatment of symptoms is fear of overdosing or harming the client.

Whereas some factors act as barriers to treatment of symptoms, other factors can facilitate caregiver treatment. Factors that facilitate treatment work by prompting the caregivers to administer a medication. Facilitating factors include receiving information on management of symptoms from a home hospice provider; instruction regarding which symptoms are more likely to occur (related to the disease and to past client experiences); ongoing interaction with the nurse and reliance on the hospice nurse's judgment; the ability of the client to verify presence of a symptom; past experience observing a specific symptom; recognition of client behavior associated with a symptom (for example, reaching for emesis basin when nauseated); and perception that the symptom indicates suffering.

It is important to note that influences on caregiver decisions to treat symptoms near death will vary in their effect among caregivers and as situations and circumstances change. It is not the simple presence or absence of a factor that will predict caregiver decisions to treat: it is the effect that a factor has on a caregiver at a certain point in time. Though knowledge of potential influences on management of symptoms is helpful in identifying potential caregiver difficulties and strengths, this knowledge is limited by its relation to the particular context of the situation and by its interaction with other influencing factors.

Pain and Symptoms of Distress at the End of Life

Most of what is known about the occurrence and treatment of symptoms near death has come from studies of clients with terminal cancer. Research has identified up to 44 symptoms known to occur near death, with pain, dyspnea, delirium, nausea, and vomiting considered the most distressing for clients to endure. Although the distinction for pain is generally made, symptoms such as dyspnea and delirium can cause suffering that is equal to or greater than some types of pain. It is therefore important that these other symptoms be included in discussions with family caregivers in the home.

Like pain, dyspnea, delirium, nausea, and vomiting can intensify, decrease, or remain the same near death. Often, these symptoms need to be treated aggressively to prevent their escalation. Effective management and control of symptoms near death can be achieved most of the time with standard medications, when the client has access to experts in palliative care. Even with optimal care, a small percentage of clients will likely have intractable symptoms that may require sedation until death.

Family caregivers of clients known to be in advanced stages of a terminal illness should have plans in place to treat symptoms of distress when a client's condition begins to decline. Some healthcare providers may avoid discussing symptoms of distress or decline, in an effort to prevent caregiver distress. However, in order to be in the best position to prevent patient suffering, it is necessary to gently inform caregivers what to look for, and what to report to the hospice nurse on call, to ensure prompt treatment. Many hospice agencies arrange for small amounts of a few medications that would likely be effective for common symptoms of distress, should symptoms occur suddenly. These medications are commonly packaged as a "**symptom relief kit**" or "comfort kit." Having these kits accessible is especially important for clients who wish to remain in their homes until death.

The medications in these kits are generally in a form that can be administered by lay caregivers to clients who are unable to swallow. For example, morphine is usually supplied as a liquid solution that can be given sublingually in the cheeks or in the **buccal mucosa** (for example, front of the lower gum line). **Lorazepam** (Ativan®) tablets, which can be given for nausea or agitation, can be crushed, mixed with a drop of water, and placed under the client's tongue. Hyoscyamine tablets or Atropine ophthalmic drops are often given orally for excessive secretions. Medications can also be **compounded** and combined with a gel, which is applied on the client's skin (for example, wrist). The medication is absorbed transdermally, and the client receives the effect from whatever medication was compounded. Medications such as lorazepam (Ativan), **diphenhydramine** (Benadryl®), and **Haloperidol** (Haldol®) are often given in this form because of the ease they allow for delivering medication to clients who are agitated. Medications that require RN administration may also be added to the kit, because most hospice agencies have an RN on call who can administer the medication if needed. Only small amounts

 Development of such kits requires collaboration among pharmacists, nurses, and physicians to determine what medications should be included and how kits should be ordered and used in practice.

of medications are placed in the kit in an effort to minimize costs while allowing treatment for a variety of symptoms. Medications in the kit generally provide 12 to 16 hours of symptom management to allow relief until additional medications can be ordered and obtained.

Table 13-1 provides an example of a home hospice symptom relief kit. Use of this kit has facilitated prompt and effective relief of symptoms for many clients, while avoiding uncomfortable and costly emergency room visits or hospitalizations. Nurses admitting clients to home hospice or palliative care programs should ideally arrange to have such kits prescribed and delivered to homes prior to the onset or intensification of a distressful symptom such as pain.

In the past, clients with terminal cancer comprised the majority of hospice home care admissions. Most recently, however, cancer diagnoses account for less than half of all hospice admissions. **Table 13-2** summarizes the various hospice admission diagnoses from 2005 research findings.

Symptom relief kits may be tailored to treat symptoms likely to occur in certain patient populations. Clients with terminal conditions such as

Table 13-1 Symptom Relief Kit

Symptom	Medication	Dosage
Unrelieved pain	Morphine sulfate solution (20 mg/mL)	0.25–0.5 mL PO/SL q 1–2 hrs PRN
Unrelieved dyspnea	Morphine sulfate solution (20 mg/mL)	0.25–0.5 mL PO/SL q 1–2 hrs PRN
Dyspnea, nausea, or agitation	Lorazepam (Ativan) 1 mg tablet	0.5–1 mg tablet q 4 hrs PRN
Nausea and vomiting	Prochlorperazine (Compazine) 25 mg/0.5 mL gel	0.5 mL gel to wrist q 8 hrs PRN
Unrelieved nausea or agitation	ABH (Ativan 1 mg + Benadryl 12.5 mg + Haldol 1 mg per 0.5 mL)	0.5 mL gel to wrist q 4 hrs PRN
Loud, wet respirations or oral secretions	Hyoscyamine tabs/liquid Atropine ophthalmic drops	0.125–0.25 mg PO/SL q 4 hrs PRN 3–5 drops PO/SL q 4 hrs PRN

PO, by mouth; PRN, as needed; q, every; SL, sublingual.

Table 13-2 Diagnoses for Admission to Hospice in 2005

Diagnosis	Percent of Hospice Admissions
Cancer	46.0
Heart disease	12.0
Dementia	9.0
Debility	9.2
Lung disease	7.5
Other	16.3
Total	100.0

Source: National Hospice and Palliative Care Organization. (2006, November). *NHPCO's Facts and Figures—2005 Findings.* NHPCO.

end-stage heart disease, chronic obstructive pulmonary disease, Alzheimer's disease, amyotrophic lateral sclerosis, and cancer have all been shown to benefit from having these kits in the home.

Instructing Family Caregivers on Symptom Management

Before instructing family members on how to manage a client's pain or symptoms of distress near death, the nurse needs to assess the family's understanding of the situation and the family's plan regarding resuscitation and hospitalization. The nurse then instructs caregivers to ask the client if he or she is having pain, shortness of breath, nausea, or other discomfort every two hours and as needed. Ideally, the caregiver should measure the intensity of the pain or shortness of breath using a method that both the client and caregiver can easily understand and implement. The simplest method involves rating the symptom from 0 to 10, with 0 indicating no pain or shortness of breath (dyspnea) and 10 indicating the worst pain or dyspnea possible. Clients may not be able, however, to use numeric ratings to conceptualize or communicate intensity of symptoms, particularly as death nears. In these situations, caregivers need not be concerned with rating the pain but should instead focus on watching the client for any symptom of distress and medicating the client based on the presence of the distress. Family are taught to look for objective signs of pain or distress such as grimacing, moaning, restlessness, or confusion and contact the hospice nurse if they need assistance in determining what this represents. Caregivers may need to be told that they cannot rely on clients to report pain or dyspnea on their own.

Times, types, and amounts of medications administered should be written down in a diary or central log to which other family members and professional caregivers have ready access. This diary is used to evaluate the effectiveness of symptom management over time and to adjust medication schedules when necessary.

Family caregivers have described multiple uncertainties when managing medications for a client in the home, and it is known that they do not administer as-needed medications as frequently as they could be used. To facilitate medication management of a client's pain, shortness of breath, or other symptoms, a plan should minimize the frequency with which caregivers are faced with decision-making and optimize the control of the symptom. Long-acting opioids often accomplish the goal of minimizing dosing and controlling pain and shortness of breath. However, long-acting opioids are not usually initiated until clients demonstrate tolerance to a certain amount of narcotic. Initially, opioids are given as short-acting doses, with an increase in frequency when needed. Symptoms requiring medications other than opioids are also treated with short-acting doses of medications as needed. It may be prudent, however, to have family caregivers administer medications for any symptom on an around-the-clock schedule to facilitate better symptom control. For example, clients who begin to have shortness of breath may be scheduled to receive immediate-release morphine sulfate 5 mg SL every 2 hours around-the-clock, as opposed to every 2 hours PRN.

It is known that family caregivers committed to a client's comfort until death can effectively manage medications for a dying person's pain in the home. Family caregivers, however, report that they need the information and ongoing clinical support that an expert in end-of-life care (for example, hospice nurse) provides to accomplish this. Caregivers rely on the assistance of a hospice nurse when they initially become involved in the management of pain in the home. Caregivers have also stated that they rely on the ongoing assessments and reinforcement of instructions related to administering medications that the nurse provides on visits to the home throughout the dying process. The interaction with the hospice nurse on each visit provides caregivers with the reassurance that they are making accurate assessments and giving appropriate care. It is important that family believe they have provided safe, effective care to their loved ones not only during the period of symptom management, but also after the client's death. The experience of managing a person's pain near death is a process that continues to be experienced even after the client's death.

Despite having administered safe amounts of analgesic to promote comfort, family caregivers have reported that they sometimes experience guilt when they reflect on their medication management of symptoms, even after the client's death. This experience of guilt is likely to occur when caregivers have been in the role of managing medications for a short period of time and/or when the client died soon after the caregiver administered morphine.

The nurse should request medications (and routes) that are most conducive to the caregivers' abilities. For example, family caregivers may express aversion to and perceived difficulty in administering rectal suppositories. Some family caregivers, however, may be open to learning and using this route. Clients may also have an aversion to the rectal route, although the assumption that all clients have this aversion should not be made. Some clients may actually prefer the rectal route, for example, if oral medications cause nausea. Intramuscular or subcutaneous injections are generally avoided in clients at the end of life because of the pain they inflict.

Strategies to help identify barriers or facilitating factors for treatment of symptoms include assessing caregivers for fears, conflicts, their perception of symptoms related to suffering, and past client perceptions of medications. The hospice nurse should instruct caregivers regarding which symptoms of distress are most likely to occur based on the client's diagnosis and past symptoms. The hospice nurse should also offer daily visits to clients experiencing changes in symptoms and/or changes in treatment. Clients with stable symptoms should be offered a hospice RN visit at least every two days to assess clients for symptoms, review medication management plans, and verify medication plans with caregivers. Even caregivers who verbalize understanding of medication management of symptoms state that they welcome the reassurance that the hospice nurse can give them. They appreciate knowing that their loved one is comfortable and that symptoms are being managed well. Caregivers are encouraged to call the hospice RN on call if they have any concerns or questions. Phone access to a hospice registered nurse 24-hours-a-day is provided by most home hospice agencies.

CASE STUDY RESOLVED

During her initial visit to M. B.'s home, the nurse assessed that M. B.'s mother would be the primary caregiver and manager of medications, but that she was only in this role during the day. The nurse observed that M. B. was experiencing pain and nausea, and that she had a short episode of dyspnea on exertion. The nurse verified that the family was aware that M. B. was near death and discussed the goals of comfort until death at home, with no resuscitation. After reviewing and verifying that M. B.'s mother and her husband were able to identify the medications in the home for nausea, pain, and/or shortness of breath, the nurse demonstrated how to administer each one. She administered a 25 mg prochlorperazine suppository, which was prescribed PRN for nausea or vomiting. Although M. B. had been taking Percocet for pain, her pain was not well controlled. The nurse suggested that M. B. try the liquid morphine sulfate. Morphine sulfate in its elixir form is easier for the patient to swallow, easier to administer than a pill, and easy to titrate. The nurse administered the liquid morphine sublingually in the client's cheek (buccal mucosa). Within 15 minutes, M. B.'s pain and nausea were greatly relieved.

Recognizing that the nausea and pain would likely recur if medications were not routinely administered, the nurse developed a medication plan in writing to include administration of a prochlorperazine antiemetic suppository at least every 8 hours, and analgesia (liquid morphine sulfate 10 mg) at least every 3 hours. Based on M. B.'s diagnosis of lung cancer and her dyspnea with activity, the nurse knew that she was at risk for having shortness of breath/dyspnea occur as death neared. To further assess the risk, the nurse auscultated M. B.'s lungs and assessed for other symptoms of fluid volume excess such as edema. Because her lungs were clear and M. B. denied shortness of breath at rest, the nurse did not include more scheduled medication for dyspnea other than the liquid morphine sulfate, which works well for both pain and dyspnea.

Noting that M. B.'s mother would be leaving and her husband would likely assume the caregiver role, the nurse turned her attention to the husband. She recognized that he was afraid and anxious based on his statements, "I don't think I can do this." The husband also stated "I cannot give a suppository." Recognizing that the husband also wanted to fulfill his wife's request to die at home, the nurse asked M. B.'s mother if there was any family member or friend that could stop by the house briefly at 10 PM to administer another suppository. M. B.'s sister was contacted and agreed to do this. M. B.'s husband said that he could give the morphine solution, and her mother stated she would give the next scheduled antiemetic suppository when she returned in the morning.

Recognizing that suppositories are difficult for many family members to administer, the nurse called the physician and requested an order for the symptom relief kit, which was prepared especially for hospice patients, with compounded medications in gel forms for nausea, vomiting, anxiety, and restlessness. A telephone call was made to the compounding pharmacy to arrange for the kit to be delivered in the morning.

To minimize M. B.'s pain and dyspnea with activity, the nurse offered to insert a Foley catheter, to which the client agreed. A home health aide was assigned to visit the client early each morning, and she agreed to assume most of the catheter care. The nurse eliminated medications that were no longer necessary for symptom management, repeated instructions regarding the scheduled medications for nausea and pain, and instructed the family that one extra dose of morphine solution could be given hourly if needed for pain or shortness of breath. The husband and mother were instructed to call hospice if pain, nausea, or dyspnea were not relieved by the medications, and/or if the client became agitated, restless, or exhibited other symptoms of distress. The nurse assured the husband that hospice was only a phone call away and encouraged him to take one day at a time. The nurse also stated she would phone the husband later that evening to assess how things were going and that she would return that evening if needed.

Because M. B. was actively dying and was at risk for increased intensity of her pain, nausea, and dyspnea, a hospice nurse visited M. B. each day to assess her symptoms, the effectiveness of the medication plan, and how the family was coping. The nurse visited M. B. in the morning for this purpose, and to instruct the family on the symptom relief kit. Given the fact that administering the prochlorperazine suppository required extra effort from family not living in the home, the nurse recommended that the prochlorperazine compounded gel for nausea in the symptom relief kit be substituted for the prochlorperazine suppository. With the physician's approval, the prochlorperazine suppository was discontinued, and M. B. was started on the prochlorperazine gel from the kit. Having received morphine sulfate 0.5 mL three times during the night, M. B. had no signs or symptoms of pain, discomfort, or shortness of breath.

Two days after her admission to home hospice, M. B. started grimacing and moaning, especially when turned in bed, and she had labored breathing. Morphine sulfate elixir 0.5 mL given every hour was effective in resolving the moaning, grimacing, and labored breathing. In an effort to better manage the discomfort and labored breathing, the nurse obtained a physician's approval to begin a 6.25 mg fentanyl (Duragesic) patch. The patch was meant to take the place of the morphine sulfate elixir. Because the patch does not provide therapeutic effect for 12–17 hours, the caregivers were instructed to continue to give morphine sulfate every 1 to 2 hours if needed. On day three, M. B. appeared comfortable, without grimacing, moaning, or shortness of breath, with only occasional morphine sulfate elixir.

Two days later, M. B. became very restless and agitated. To rule out the possibility that pain was the cause of the agitation, three doses of morphine sulfate where given, but there was no improvement. Because the pain had been well controlled, it was thought that the restlessness likely represented the **delirium** seen with **terminal agitation**.

Terminal agitation is an observable syndrome characterized by inability to rest, occurring in clients with varying diagnoses during the last days of life.

M. B. was given a 1 mg lorazepam (Ativan) tablet, crushed and mixed with a drop of water, under her tongue (physician orders to give this medication were in the symptom relief kit). M. B.'s agitation improved for approximately 2 hours, but she became agitated again. The hospice nurse instructed the family to apply 0.5 mL of the **Ativan/Benadryl/Haldol (ABH)** gel, which was effective. The medication management plan was revised to include administration of 0.5 mL gel every 4 hours around-the-clock, with lorazepam (Ativan) 1 mg crushed and given sublingually every 4 hours PRN.

With careful planning involving the hospice team, the medication schedule for M. B. was maintained, and her nausea, pain, and agitation were well controlled. She died peacefully two days later in her home.

CHAPTER 13 • REVIEW QUESTIONS

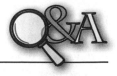

1. Your client, who is actively dying, is groaning and moaning. Your priority at this time is to assess for:
    A. Fatigue
    B. Hunger
    C. Pain
    D. Shortness of breath.

2. In the home, family caregivers assume most of the responsibility for treating a dying person's pain. A factor that would prompt family caregivers to administer a medication for pain would be:
    A. Utilization of rectal route
    B. Fear of overdosing the patient
    C. The client's inability to speak
    D. The perception that the person is suffering

3. What is the purpose of logging the times and amounts of medications given to a client near death?
    A. To evaluate the competency of family caregivers
    B. To identify substance abuse
    C. To assess for potential overdosing of medications
    D. To help in evaluating the effectiveness of symptom management

4. Which of the following medications is most appropriate for treatment of terminal agitation:
    A. Atropine ophthalmic drops
    B. Morphine sulfate
    C. Ativan/Benadryl/Haldol
    D. hyoscyamine

ANSWERS AND RATIONALES

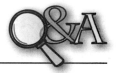

1. **C.** There are multiple causes of restlessness and agitation near the end of life. The healthcare provider often administers an analgesic to help determine if pain is the cause of the restlessness. Resolution of the agitation supports the premise that pain was the cause.

2. **D.** Research shows that family caregivers' perception that a symptom indicates suffering will be a facilitating factor to their administering medication. Barriers to treatment include the client's inability to report the symptom and fear of overdosing or harming the client. Some family caregivers have an aversion to using the rectal route to administer medications.

3. **D.** Although family caregivers have demonstrated commitment to clients' comfort near death, they do not administer as-needed medications as frequently as they could be given. They should not, however, be evaluated in terms of their competency. Healthcare providers should recognize that family caregivers can be effective in management of medications despite their uncertainties, fears that they will overmedicate, and their lack of clinical decision-making abilities. Family caregivers are asked to keep a log or diary of the times, types, and amounts of medication given to evaluate the effectiveness of the symptom management plan.

4. **C.** The combined effects of Ativan/Benadryl/Haldol are often effective for terminal agitation. Atropine ophthalmic drops given orally are used to dry up secretions. Morphine sulfate is used for pain or dyspnea. Morphine would be appropriate for treatment of agitation if pain were the etiology. Hyoscyamine is given for secretions.

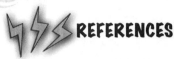

REFERENCES

Emanuel, L., Ferris, F. D., von Gunten, C. F., & von Roenn, J. H. (2006, August 28). The last hours of living: practical advice for clinicians. *Medscape*. Available from www.medscape.com.

Given, B., & Given, C. (1994). Family home care for individuals with cancer. *Oncology, 8*(5), 77–93.

Kazanowski, M. (2006). Symptom management in palliative care. In M. Matzo & D. Sherman (Eds.), *Palliative Care Nursing* (pp. 319–344). New York: Springer.

Kazanowski, M. (1998). *Commitment to the end: Family caregivers' medication management of symptoms in patients with cancer near death.* PhD dissertation, Graduate School of Nursing, Boston College, Chestnut Hill, MA.

National Hospice and Palliative Care Organization. (2006, November). *NHPCO's Facts and Figures—2005 Findings.* Retrieved September 27, 2007, from www.nhpco.org/files/public/2005-facts-and-figures.pdf.

Steele, R., & Fitch, M. (1996). Needs of family caregivers of patients receiving home hospice care for cancer. *Oncol Nurs Forum, 23,* 823–828.

Taylor, E., Ferrell, B., Grant, M., & Cheyney, L. (1993). Managing cancer pain at home: The decisions and ethical conflicts of patients, family caregivers, and homecare nurses. *Oncol Nurs Forum, 20,* 919–927.

INDEX

NOTE: *t* with page number indicates tables.